1995

ETHICS IN HEALTH
SERVICES MANAGEMENT

ETHICS IN HEALTH SERVICES MANAGEMENT
Second Edition

by

Kurt Darr, J.D., Sc.D., FACHE
Professor
Department of Health Services Management and Policy
The George Washington University
Washington, D.C.

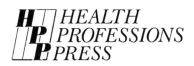

HEALTH
PROFESSIONS
PRESS

Baltimore • London • Toronto • Sydney

Health Professions Press
P.O. Box 10624
Baltimore, Maryland 21285-0624

Typeset by Brushwood Graphics, Inc., Baltimore, Maryland.
Manufactured in the United States of America by
The Maple Press, York, Pennsylvania.

Fourth printing, October 1995.

Darr, Kurt.
    Ethics in health services management   /   by Kurt Darr.—2nd ed.
        p.   cm.
    Includes bibliographical references and index.
    ISBN 1–878812–04–1
    1. Health services administration—Moral and ethical aspects.   2. Medical
ethics.   I. Title.
[DNLM: 1. Ethics, Medical.   2. Health Services—organization & administration.   W 84.1 D225e]
RA394.D35   1991
174'.2—dc20
DNLM/DLC
for Library of Congress   90–15630
                                                                           CIP

∞

CONTENTS

∞

PREFACE

THE SECOND EDITION HAS THE SAME INTENT as the first: to assist managers of health services organizations in preventing and solving administrative and biomedical ethical problems and to provide this assistance in a readily usable form. It suggests methodologies and techniques by which managers can understand, analyze, and solve ethical problems. A major collateral purpose is to encourage and aid managers to develop and hone a personal ethic.

To encourage initial reading and facilitate later use as a reference, brevity has been a major criterion. The text seeks to inform users about ethical issues and potential problems so that they may be solved knowledgeably and effectively. Extensive use is made of case examples that are based on situations reported in the popular press and professional literature, or known from the author's personal experience. The use of case studies should help the reader learn to apply the principles.

As with all management problems, there are few, if any, ready answers to ethical problems, and no attempt is made to provide them here. "Cookbook" approaches lack feasibility in virtually all problem-solving activity because nuances of fact, setting, and personality vary with each situation. The approach here is to provide information, examples, and analyses useful to developing the individualized solutions needed by health services organizations and their managers.

Managers address problems in an organized and logical fashion. This means identifying and analyzing the problem, developing alternative means to solve it, and formulating criteria by which to evaluate possible solutions. Implementation is critical. Evaluation must always be included—preferably built-in, rather than added as an afterthought. Evaluation provides the all-important feedback necessary to make the adjustments that enhance performance. This methodology is similar to that used in moral reasoning and management problem solving. It is a focal point of this book.

The need for ethical decision making—applied ethics—by managers in health services organizations has always existed. Development of new technologies, external pressures from government and community, and changing social mores have combined, however, to make the decision-making and implementation processes more critical, and to impose harsher penalties on those who ignore their implications.

The book is organized into five parts. Part I describes various moral philosophies and moral principles, and examines the ways in which managers approach ethical problems. Part II examines administrative procedures for effecting ethical decision making. Part III provides an in-depth look at administrative ethical issues commonly found in health services organizations. Part IV examines biomedical ethical issues. Part V analyzes the emerging ethical issues raised by competition and AIDS.

The first edition was a book that I had long wanted to write. As technology has extended life and death, as demands for health care and services continue to exceed resources, and as economic and competitive pressures buffet health services organizations, their managers will increasingly be major actors in a complex drama. If this second edition assists managers to identify, analyze, and solve ethical problems more effectively, I will have achieved a major goal.

∞

ACKNOWLEDGMENTS

THE IDEA FOR THIS BOOK DATES TO the late 1970s, but it was not until the first edition was published in 1987 that it achieved fruition. Those who were instrumental in preparing the first edition have my continuing thanks.

Robert G. Shouldice, D.B.A., kindly advised me on the managed care section, and I thank him for his efforts. Richard F. Southby, Ph.D., Chairman of the Department of Health Services Management and Policy at The George Washington University, has in all ways supported my research and publishing efforts. His encouragement greatly facilitated my work; for that I am most grateful. Ben Burdetsky, Ph.D., Dean of The George Washington University School of Business and Public Management, has nurtured an environment in which productive research and writing activities are encouraged, and I appreciate his efforts.

My production editor, Barbara S. Karni, improved the manuscript in a great many ways, and I thank her for her fine work.

Research and other assistance were provided by Laurie Farrington and Shelby Higgins. They worked diligently, often under significant time constraints. I am very appreciative of their efforts, and I wish them every success in their careers in health services management.

ANNE
Still lighting the way

∞

INTRODUCTION

Two themes underlie this book: the autonomy, primacy, and protection of the patient*; and the role of the health services manager as a moral agent who leads the health services organization.

This book seeks to help health services managers develop a personal ethic and gain a basic understanding of administrative and biomedical ethical issues, and suggests a methodology for solving the problems these issues raise. The emphasis is on normative ethics (the study of what should be done). Some attention is paid to descriptive ethics (the study of what is actually done) and on metaethics (the study of ethical systems) because they assist in understanding normative ethics. Theories of ethical relativism and ethical nihilism are not addressed. Ethical relativism states that there are no absolute truths, and that all answers to ethical questions are equally right or morally correct, depending on a culture's viewpoint. Nihilists consider no choice correct. In a sense, both theories are similar, and neither helps meet the needs of patients, staff, or organization. Nor do these theories assist managers who have the difficult task of solving ethical problems. Furthermore, relativist and nihilist perspectives are of little value in helping the manager formulate a personal ethic.

For the health services manager, a personal ethic is a moral framework within which the appropriate relationship with employees, patients, organization, and community develops. In this regard, the manager is not, and cannot be, a morally neutral technocrat. The manager is a moral agent—someone who morally affects and is morally affected by actions taken. This means that management decision making is not value free; in a moral sense, it affects its environment and all touched by it.

The patient looks to the organization and those working in it to perform services that are unique in society. Managers' responsibilities to their patients take precedence over their fiduciary responsibilities to their organizations. Protecting the patient means more than providing safe surroundings and competent

---

*For ease of reading, *patient* is used to describe anyone served by a health services organization.

1

staff. It means more than accreditation by the Joint Commission on Accreditation of Healthcare Organizations. It means more than showing a surplus on the financial statement. The manager is the organization's conscience. This duty is exemplified by the organization's willingness, prompted and led by its management, to recognize the inherent human dignity of the patient, and to do so through effective programs that make this recognition a reality. It means using appropriate consent forms and procedures, and aggressively ascertaining that all persons who have contact with patients are fully qualified and use their qualifications to serve the patient. It means not treating the patient as an adversary, and not deserting the patient should something go wrong during treatment. If the organization has honestly and forthrightly done its best, it can face the consequences of an error without shame, do whatever it can to mitigate the injury, and work out an equitable solution. The loop is closed when the organization, under management's direction, determines the cause of the problem, and develops and implements means to minimize or prevent its recurrence.

When treating a patient, physicians must respect the decisions made by that patient (or as appropriate, a proxy). There will be times, however, when the principle of justice requires that a prospective decision process include criteria of cost–benefit analysis and utilitarianism (the greatest good for the greatest number). Even here, though, the organization recognizes the human dignity and worth of persons who as yet are unserved, or only partially served.

How does the health services organization develop and implement a just policy? How does it strive to treat its patients as equals, and to work with patients to serve their interests? Implementation of a just policy begins with the organization's philosophy, which should explictly state the nature of the relationship between the patient and the organization. This philosophy should reflect the view that the patient is autonomous, and is entitled to be treated with respect and dignity. In a real sense, it is based on a contract—an implicit, but verifiable understanding between patient and provider that is grounded in mutual trust and confidence. It recognizes that whenever possible, patients should retain control of their lives.

Once recognized in that basic statement, the organization's philosophy, the relationship with patients must be reflected in all derivative mission statements, policies, procedures, and rules, but especially in all relationships with patients and community. If not operationalized, the organization will be judged cynical about itself and those it serves. This cynicism is readily recognized by staff, and is likely to be reflected in how patients are treated. Although most of the staff will not succumb to the negative implications of this inconsistency, it will be an underlying, festering incongruity.

A major participant in developing and maintaining the appropriate relationship is the physician—necessarily a prime actor. The role of physician and organization are complementary, but the organization remains morally (ethically) and legally accountable for the physician's activities.

CONCERN ABOUT ETHICS

Ethics is a word used with increasing frequency everywhere in health care. Daily, questions are asked about making the ethically right choice. Seemingly straightforward and value-free management decisions have ethical implications for patients, staff, organization, community, or society. Many decisions that cause ethical dilemmas are the result of the continuing revolutions in biology and technology that began several decades ago. Fiscal constraints and cost cutting exacerbate existing ethical problems and raise new ones. Beyond these causes is the enhanced level of awareness resulting from the research and writing of ethicists and the work of government commissions on experimentation and bioethics.

Ethical dilemmas occur when decision makers are drawn in two directions by competing courses of action that are based on different moral philosophies, different organizational philosophies, conflicting duties, or an ill-defined sense of right and wrong. For example, staff members may be asked to follow rules they consider inappropriate or unjust, or two moral principles may conflict with one another. A nurse's duty to preserve life, for example, clashes with the duty to serve the patient and the patient's wishes not to be kept alive by applying artificial means. Another source of ethical dilemma is the existence of two compelling, defensible positions on an issue, such as the possible conception of a genetically defective infant. Required genetic screening and counseling for those at risk clearly conflict with the primacy of individual autonomy. Conclusions vary when decision makers place different weights on various considerations, such as the importance of personal liberty or privacy. Ethical decisions are also affected by whether or not the economic and/or political implications for society are considered. For some ethical issues, one can conclude that reasonable persons could differ as to the "right" result. For the overwhelming majority of ethical issues, however, one answer clearly emerges as morally superior to the others.

Beyond biomedical ethical problems, some of which become "dilemmas" and receive great media attention, there is the important need to identify and solve management problems with ethical dimensions. These administrative ethical problems do not as frequently represent competing, ethically defensible choices. Solving them is usually a matter of recognition and resolve—doing what is ethically correct.

Are laws and regulations the problem or the solution? Some observers may perceive that ethical dilemmas exist because laws or regulations external to the organization fail to guide action clearly. Others may perceive that the presence of laws forces organizations and managers to act in specific ways, thus causing ethical problems. Depending on the issue and facts, both views may be correct. Even when external rules are present, the decision maker must decide when they apply, how they should be interpreted, and whether they should be obeyed at all. In fact, by designating and clarifying rules, there will be less middle ground, and the problems will be even starker and more difficult to solve. Some may even choose to ignore the rules and apply personal standards. Others will apply rules dogmatically, and choose not to think about the underlying philosophical or ethical issues that are raised. Conversely, some ethical problems result because no established external rules or regulations assist decision makers. For some issues, ethical problems have developed more quickly than the ability of the health services field or society to solve them. For others, there is a lack of consensus as to what the rule should be.

DEFINING ETHICS

Defining *ethics* precisely is difficult, because it has a variety of meanings. For philosophers, ethics is the formal study of morality. Sociologists see ethics as the mores, customs, and behavior found in a culture. For physicians, it means meeting the expectations of a profession and society, and acting in certain ways toward patients. Health services managers should view ethics as a special charge and a responsibility to the patient, to the organization and its personnel, to themselves and the profession, and ultimately, but less directly, to society.

Distinctions are commonly blurred, but ethical problems may be divided into administrative and biomedical problems. Administrative ethical problems involve the manager and the profession, the organization, the patient, or society. Biomedical ethical problems involve individuals or identified groups of patients in their relationships with providers, organizations, or each other. Depending on the issue, the manager is usually involved less directly in biomedical ethical problems.

The word *dilemma* is commonly used to describe ethical problems, because it emphasizes the difficulty of finding the morally correct solution. Ethical problems are often difficult to solve, but few are appropriately labeled dilemmas.

SOURCES OF LAW

Because of the dynamic relationship between law and ethics (morality), it is useful to begin a book about ethics by reviewing briefly the development of law. Every organized society has a code or system of laws that distinguishes acceptable from unacceptable behavior, and establishes penalties for transgressors. Law may be defined simply as a sytem of principles and rules of human conduct prescribed or recognized by a supreme authority. This definition includes both criminal and civil law. Ethics is the study of standards of conduct and moral judgment. When referring to a profession, it is the system or code of morals that guides that group.

In its moral underpinnings, criminal law is especially clear in reflecting society's sense of right and wrong—its ethics (morality). In a democratic society, laws can be said to be derived from and reflect the views of justice and fairness held by the majority of the population. This is less true in civil law, which governs relations among individuals and includes contracts and commercial transactions. Here, greater emphasis is put on predictability, stability, and property rights.

Some societies regarded the law as a gift from the gods. Plato's *Republic* postulated the ideal state as one based on rational order and ruled by philosopher kings. Plato considered written law a regrettable oversimplification that could not take into account all the differences and conditions in parties and situations involved in legal disputes. He believed that the best situation was one in which a philosopher could apply an unwritten law. When his own experience proved this impossible, he accepted a written law administered by authorities without regard to circumstances of the persons involved.[1] Thus the concept of a rule of law, not of men, became established in Anglo-American legal tradition. However, because of the absurd results that can occur when civil law is applied without considering the situations of the concerned parties, the concept of unwritten law preferred by Plato was continued in only a limited fashion. At common law, parallel court systems developed, and actions in civil matters could be brought in either court system. In some states, courts of equity hear cases in which fairness is the primary concern. Most states, however, have combined actions at law and equity into one system.

Democratically derived legislative enactments tend to reflect societal views about morality: which acts are right, and which are wrong. To the extent that democratic processes represent a majority view, laws reflect the moral values of most people. Substantial minorities may have contrary views, however, and may consider the law so unjust that they risk the penalties of breaking it. An historical example is the Volstead Act, which instituted prohibition by amending the federal constitution. Violation was widespread until repeal over a decade later in 1933. Contemporary examples are the common disregard of speed limits and prohibitions against the use of marijuana.

Because of the link between societal views of right and wrong and the law, morality is reflected in all types of law, whether formal or nonformal. A leading jurisprudent, Edgar Bodenheimer, identifies formal sources of law as constitutions, statutes, executive orders, administrative regulations, ordinances, charters and bylaws of autonomous or semiautonomous bodies, treaties, and judicial precedents. Nonformal sources of law are those that have not received an authoritative, or at least articulated, formulation and embodiment in a formalized legal document. They include standards of justice, principles of reason and consideration of the nature of things (*natura rerum*), equity for individuals, public policies, moral convictions, social trends, and customary law.

Bodenheimer's inclusion of the charters and bylaws of autonomous and semiautonomous bodies in the list of formal sources of law has significance for health services management. Such documents include the articles of incorporation and bylaws of the organization. The organization's philosophy and mission statement may be included in either or both, and will appear in expanded form in other documents published by the organization. These are very important. Medical staff bylaws, rules, and regulations also reflect the organization's philosophy and mission, and must be consistent with them.

In addition to their importance in containing the philosophy and mission of the organization, such documents represent an organization's basic laws. Persons affected by the organization—employees, medical staff, patients—look to them for guidance. Parts of these laws, such as the medical staff bylaws, describe in detail the rights and obligations of the medical staff. Should a legal controversy develop, courts or other reviewing bodies look at these documents as sources of formal law.

Bodenheimer's definition of formal law is broad enough to include codes of ethics used by professional associations to distinguish acceptable from unacceptable behavior to guide members' actions. To be adequately implemented, a code must be interpreted and enforced. Such activities give guidance about a code's application and decision making, give it dynamism and life, and provide the important virtues of consistency and predictability.

RELATIONSHIP BETWEEN ETHICS AND LAW

For the professions, ethics is much more than obeying the law. The law represents only the minimum standard of morality established by society to guide interactions among its people and between the people and the government. The law governing one's relationships includes few positive duties. Only in unique situations is one person obliged to aid another, for example. The law concentrates on prohibitions—the "thou shalt nots." Professions are bound by the law, but they have a higher calling, one that includes numerous positive duties to patients and society, as well as to each other.

Positive duties are not exclusive to the professions. Individuals may view their roles in life as including a duty to aid fellow human beings, or to work on their behalf. In many respects, this positive duty means practicing the Golden Rule: "Do unto others as you would have them do unto you." This is a far more demanding relationship than merely refraining from doing something that interferes with someone else, or enacting a law that protects one person from another.

It is paradoxical that law both prevents and causes ethical problems. Absent applicable public law, managers rely on the formal law of the organization, documents such as organizational philosophy and mission statement (its ethic), and a personal ethic to guide decision making. The presence of public law may or may not be determinative in solving a problem. Whether or not public law exists, choices must be made. Even when public law is clear, ethical problems may remain. An example is the Supreme Court decision that a constitutional right of privacy prevents state and local governments from interfering in a woman's choice to have an abortion during the first trimester of pregnancy. The controversy over the morality (ethics) of abortion is intense.

Statutes and codes of ethics are formal sources of law. While statutes apply to all members of society, or to large subsets of it, however, a code of ethics affects only members of a particular group. The choice to belong to a particular group may not be completely voluntary: colleagues have certain expectations and demands; employers consider certain credentials, including memberships, important in judging qualifications; and better informed consumers ask questions and express views about an individual's memberships. Nonetheless, participation in groups that have codes is, at root, voluntary.

Licensure is common for clinical personnel in the health services field. Many health services professional groups, including certain types of managers, such as nursing facility managers, have ethical standards included in the statutes that license them. In such cases, these ethical standards have the force of law. Nevertheless, this does not relieve the professional association of the responsibility to regulate members' behavior, even to the point of adopting more stringent guidelines.

Groups whose codes of ethics are only a private statement of acceptable behavior for their members, and whose codes are not reflected in statutes or regulations, have a heavier burden of monitoring their members. If any monitoring is done, they must do it. A profession's obligation to protect society's interests substantially heightens its need to monitor its members' actions effectively. That is the hallmark of a profession.

In any disciplinary proceeding taken pursuant to a licensing statute, the actions of a public regulatory body are distinct from those of the private group. If holding a valid license is a prerequisite to belonging to a professional group, expulsion may follow delicensure, but this occurs only after a separate formal hearing and review process by the professional group.

The correspondence between law and ethics might seem to be one-to-one—anything lawful is ethical and vice versa. This need not be the case, however, for several reasons. The most important reason is that the law states the least that is expected from members of society, and as noted, contains few, if any, positive duties. Professions expect their members to comply with the law, but they often add substantially to this standard. The result is that although the law may not require a particular action, a professional's code of ethics may require it. Thus, performing (or not performing) a particular activity may be legal, but not ethical.

A model useful to show the relationship of law to ethics has been developed by Henderson and is presented in Figure 1. It suggests the succession of events leading to corporate decisions coming to public scrutiny and eventually a determination as to whether they are legal and/or ethical. It is necessarily an *ex*

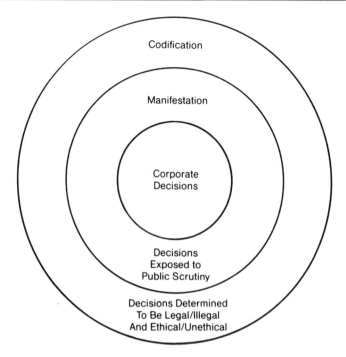

Figure 1. The relationship between law and ethics. (From Henderson, V.E. [1982]. The ethical side of enterprise. *Sloan Management Review, 23*, pp. 37–47. Copyright © 1982 by the Sloan Management Review Association. All rights reserved. Reprinted by permission.)

post facto judgment, despite attempts by management to predict consequences of a decision. This model suggests that for many corporate actions, it cannot be known with certainty whether those who eventually judge the decision will consider it legal (determined by law enforcement officials) or ethical (determined by the profession or the general public). This adds a high degree of uncertainty to decision making inside and outside the health services system. It is usually easier to predict whether an action will be deemed legal than it is to predict whether an action will be judged ethical.

Figure 2 is a matrix of the combinations of legal, illegal, ethical, and unethical. In Quadrant I, managers are acting legally and ethically.

Quadrant II contains decisions that are ethical, but illegal. The American College of Healthcare Executives' Code of Ethics makes unethical the commission of any illegal acts. Given this broad prohibition, it would be difficult, if not impossible, for health services managers to justify as ethical an act that is illegal.

Quadrant III includes decisions that are unethical, but legal, and applies the concept that ethical standards, especially those of a profession, hold the member to a higher standard than does the law. Examples include failing to take

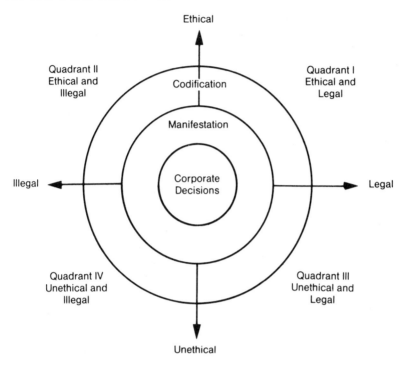

Figure 2. A matrix of possible outcomes concerning the ethics and legality of corporate decisions. (From Henderson, V.E. [1982]. The ethical side of enterprise. *Sloan Management Review*, *23*, pp. 37–47. Copyright © 1982 by the Sloan Management Review Association. All rights reserved. Reprinted by permission.)

reasonable steps to protect the patient from medical malpractice, and manager self-aggrandizement at the expense of patients.

Quadrant IV includes activities that are illegal and unethical. Embezzlement would fall in this quadrant, as would failing to meet local fire safety requirements or filing false Medicare or Medicaid reports.

CONCLUSION

It is important to stress that there is a dynamic between law and ethics—each affects and is affected by the other. Professional codes and conduct reflect society's perceptions of a profession, as well as that profession's perceptions of itself. To the extent that the law reflects society's need to protect itself and regulate conduct, licensure laws provide further clarification of what is expected of a professional group. The morality reflected in the law evolves, but is likely to lag behind private morality and ethics. In this regard, the law leads some subsets of society, but follows others.

Contemporary demands on health services organizations and managers may seem inconsistent in many ways with the often idealized statements found in codes of ethics. Managers must recognize their responsibility, however, and strive to transform the ideal into reality. Managers see themselves and are seen by others as moral agents who have a critical role in the organization and its efforts to serve, protect, and further the interests of patient and community.

Gandhi said that noncooperation with evil is as much a duty as cooperation with good. Edmund Burke said that the only thing necessary for the triumph of evil is that good men do nothing. Both philosophies are germane to the health services field, especially for its managers. Understanding their ethical obligations and meeting the imperatives these obligations provide are essential.

If the findings of a Gallup poll about corporate ethics are applicable to the health services field, we are confronted by a major challenge. That poll showed that 30% of the general public believes corporate ethics are slipping; 25% of middle-level executives agree.

> The poll focused on unethical personal behavior in the workplace. Over three quarters of the executives interviewed use company phones to make personal long-distance calls. Almost as many take home office supplies. Thirty-five per cent say that they have somewhat overstated deductions on their tax forms. And 80 per cent have driven while drunk. One financial services executive offered a list of unethical practices that included "bribes, falsifying documents, improper financial statements, bid rigging, and price collusion."
>
> What determines a person's ethics in the workplace? Age, for one thing. In the Gallup poll, younger executives consistently behaved less ethically. Education also influenced responses—negatively. A far higher proportion of college graduates than those without high school diplomas took home office supplies and called in sick when they were not.[2]

If ethical problems among managers in business are extensive, it is likely that the problem has touched the health services field as well. The examples of unethical behavior found in the Gallup poll focus on the relationship between the manager and the organization. What about the manager's relationship with those served by the organization? Managing health services organizations will always be among the most demanding work in society. No one said it would be easy; few in the field expect kudos for their service. But we raise the pride of profession and self, and fulfill our role if we view ourselves as moral agents whose primary duty is to protect our patients' interests and further their care. This is the challenge of health services management.

NOTES

1. Edgar Bodenheimer, *Jurisprudence: The Philosophy and Method of the Law* (Cambridge: Harvard University Press, 1974), 6.
2. "In Search of the Honest Executive: A View from the Top and the Middle," *Hastings Center Report 14* (February 1984): 2.

I

∞

IDENTIFYING AND SOLVING ETHICAL PROBLEMS

This FIRST PART MAY BE THE MOST important in the book. The two chapters here present information basic to understanding, analyzing, and solving administrative and biomedical ethical problems. A generic background and methodology are developed and applied to a case. Although the nature of ethical problems will change over time as a result of changes in technology, the law, and financing, the framework and process developed here will remain useful for managers.

Chapter 1 identifies and discusses moral philosophies and derivative principles—a background necessary to analyzing administrative and biomedical ethical problems. This background is critical to developing a personal ethic.

Developing problem-solving skills is an important part of educating managers. Thus, managers bring an understanding of how to solve ethical problems to this discussion of moral philosophies and derivative principles. The purpose of Chapter 2 is to build on a generic skill already in the ken of most managers. The problem-solving techniques suggested have been modified for ethical issues, but they will be very familiar to managers.

Solving biomedical ethical problems cannot be the exclusive province of physicians, nor can administrative ethics be a concern only of managers. Meeting the ethical imperative of an organization is vital, and should be part of any measure of how successfully it has met its mission and objectives. Managers must participate fully if ethical problems are to be solved effectively. Managers who behave only as technocrats ignore their responsibilities as moral agents. Applying ethical principles is too important a task to be left to others.

1

∞

MORAL PHILOSOPHIES
AND PRINCIPLES

WHAT ARE THE SOURCES OF ETHICAL guidelines? How do they help us identify and act on the morally correct choice? Philosophers, theologians, and others have grappled with these questions. In medicine, this tradition goes back to the ancient Greeks. More recently, managers and nurses have formally sought to clarify, establish, and, sometimes, enforce ethical standards. Their codes and activities usually incorporate philosophies about the appropriate relationship of providers to one another, to patients, and to society. For managers, the appropriate relationship with the organization is an additional dimension, and is included in their codes.

A natural starting point for discussing ethics and understanding how to resolve ethical problems is to review several basic moral philosophies that have heavily influenced Western European culture and thought. Among the most prominent are Kantian deontology, utilitarian teleology, natural law as developed by Thomas Aquinas, and the work of a contemporary American philosopher, John Rawls. These moral philosophies allow us to derive ethical principles, principles that should form the moral (ethical) underpinnings for delivery of health services by organizations. Furthermore, these principles guide actions and can assist managers (and other health providers) in developing a personal ethic. These operative principles are *respect for persons, beneficence, nonmaleficence, and justice.*

A case example highlights the moral philosophies and derivative principles.

Baby Boy Doe

In 1970, a male infant born at a major East Coast medical center was diagnosed as having mental retardation and duodenal atresia (the absence of a connection between the stomach and intestine). Surgeons determined that although the baby was very small, the atresia was operable, with a high probability of success. The surgery would not affect the baby's mental retardation, but would permit him to take nourishment by mouth and lead a normal life.

The parents decided to forego the surgery—something they had the legal right to do—and over the next 2 weeks the infant was left to die through dehydration and starvation. No basic determination of the extent of mental impairment had been made, nor could it have been, at the time the infant died. No attempt was made by hospital personnel or state family and social service to come to the infant's aid.

This case sends a cold shudder through most people. But feelings are insufficient. If managers are to be effective in addressing and solving—or, preferably, preventing—such problems, they must identify and understand the issues involved and the roles of the staff and the organization, and seek to apply principles of ethical conduct. In the next several sections, the moral philosophies and ethical principles involved in the Baby Boy Doe case are discussed. The case itself is then analyzed.

MORAL PHILOSOPHIES

Utilitarianism

Utilitarians are consequentialists; they evaluate an action in terms of its effect. They are teleologists, a word taken from the Greek word *telos,* meaning end. Utilitarianism has historical connections to hedonism (Epicureanism), which measured morality by the amount of pleasure obtained from an act or rule. This theory was refined by two nineteenth-century philosophers, Jeremy Bentham and John Stuart Mill. The most complete elaboration of utilitarianism was put forth by Mill. Unlike Bentham, Mill sought to distinguish pleasures (the good) on qualitative grounds. Questions about the superiority of certain pleasures, such as listening to a piano concerto, were to be answered by consulting a person of sensitivity and broad experience. (The need for such judgments somewhat diminishes the objectivity of utilitarianism.)

Mill stressed the importance of individual freedom. In *On Liberty,* he noted that freedom is a prerequisite to producing happiness, and that this makes it unacceptable for the privacy of any group or individual to be infringed in significant ways.

In selecting the morally correct option, utilitarians ignore the means of achieving an end and judge the results of an action by comparing the good brought about by a particular action to the good brought about by alternatives, or the amount of evil avoided. A modified form of utility theory is the basis for cost–benefit analysis, commonly used by economists and managers. "The greatest good for the greatest number," and "the end justifies the means"—both statements attributable to utilitarians—are merely crude gauges of utilitarianism, and cannot be applied without qualification.

Utilitarianism is divided into *act utility* and *rule utility.* Both measure consequences, and the action that brings into being the most good (understood in a nonmoral sense) is deemed the morally correct choice.

The act utilitarian judges each action independently, without reference to preestablished guidelines (rules). The amount of good, or (nonmoral) value, brought into being, and the amount of evil, or (nonmoral) disvalue, avoided by acting on a particular choice are measured. Each person affected is counted equally. This seems to give a strong sense of objectivity to this moral philosophy. Because of its episodic nature, act utilitarianism is incompatible with efforts to develop and derive the ethical principles that are a necessary part of codes of ethics and a personal ethic. Therefore, it will not receive further attention.

The rule utilitarian is also concerned only with consequences, but has prospectively considered various actions and the amount of good or evil brought into being by each. Based on these assessments, the rule utilitarian develops rules (guidelines) for action, because it has been determined that, on average, particular rules produce the most good and least evil. Therefore, these rules represent the morally correct choice. These rules are followed for all similar situations, even though for some situations they may not represent the best course of action. The rule directs selection of the morally correct choice. Rule utilitarianism is useful in developing moral principles applicable in health services management.

Deontology

Deontologists advocate a formalist approach to moral philosophy. In Greek, *deon* means duty. The foremost proponent of deontology was Immanuel Kant, an eighteenth century German philosopher. Kant's basic precept was that relations with others are based on duty. An action is moral if it arises solely from the "good will" and not from other motives. For Kant, good will is that which is good without qualification. Unlike the utilitarians, deontologists view the end as unimportant, because, in Kant's view, persons have duties to one another as moral agents, and these duties take precedence over the consequences of any actions. Kantians hold that there are certain absolute duties always in force. Among the most important duty is that of respect—"do unto others as you would have them do unto you." Kant argued that all persons have a duty in this regard; respect toward others must always be paid.

Actions taken in light of this duty must first be tested in a special fashion. Kant termed this test the *categorical imperative*. The categorical imperative requires that actions under consideration be universalized. In other words, if a principle of action is thought to be appropriate, a determination is made as to whether it can be consistently applied to all persons in all places at all times. No exceptions can be made, nor are any allowances permitted for special circumstances. If the action under consideration meets this test, it can be accepted as a duty. It fails to meet the test if it is contradictory to the overriding principle that all persons must be treated as moral equals and are, therefore, entitled to respect. Truth telling is a prominent example of a duty that meets the categorical imperative.

For the Kantian deontologist, it is logically inconsistent to argue that the terminally ill person should be euthanized, because this amounts to the self-contradictory principle that life can be improved by ending it. Similarly, caregivers should not be permitted to lie to their patients when that makes health care delivery more efficient, since such a policy would fail the test of the categorical imperative because it treats patients as means, rather than moral equals. The Golden Rule is the best shorthand statement of Kant's philosophy. Thus, in Kantian deontology, no consideration is paid to results or consequences. This does not mean that the manager must be unaware of the consequences of an action, but such consequences are not included or weighted in the ethical decision-making process.

Natural Law

Kant rejected all ethical theories based on desire or inclination; Mill defined morally right actions in terms of the happiness, or nonmoral value, produced. Unlike either Mill or Kant, natural law theorists contend that ethics must be based on a concern for the human good. They also contend that the good cannot be defined simply in terms of subjective inclinations. Rather, there is a good for human beings that is objectively desirable, although not reducible to desire.[1] Natural law is based on the view that divine law has acted to inscribe certain potentialities in all things, and these constitute the good of those things. In this sense, the theory is teleological, because it is concerned with ends. The natural law is based on Aristotelian thought as interpreted and synthesized with Christian dogma by St. Thomas Aquinas (1226–1274).[2]

The potentiality of mankind is based on that uniquely human trait, the ability to reason. According to natural law, ethics is based on the premise that man will do what is rational, and that this rationality will cause man to tend to do good and avoid evil. Natural law presumes a natural order in relationships and a predisposition by rational persons to do or refrain from doing certain things. Our ability for rational thought enables us to discover what we should do. In that effort we are guided by a partial notion of God's divine plan that is linked to our capacity for rational thought. Since natural law guides what rational man does, it serves as a basis for positive law, some of which is reflected in statutes. Our natural inclination directs us to preserve our lives and to do such rational things as avoid danger, act in self-defense, and seek medical attention when needed. Because of the ability to reason, we also see that other human beings are like us, and are therefore entitled to the same respect and dignity that we seek. A summary statement of the basic precepts of natural law is "do good and avoid evil." Applying the principles of natural law, theologians have developed a number of moral guidelines about medical services that are described in later chapters.

John Rawls

A contemporary moral philosopher, John Rawls, provides a hybrid theory of ethics that has applications in health services delivery and allocation. His theory utilizes an elaborate strategy in which all persons are behind a veil of ignorance. Persons in a hypothetical "original position" are rational and act in their own self-interest, but know nothing of their individual talents, intelligence, social and economic situation, or the like. Rawls argues that persons in such a position will identify certain principles of justice. First, all persons should have equal rights to the most extensive basic liberty compatible with similar liberty for others (the *liberty principle*). Second, social and economic inequalities should be arranged so that they are both reasonably expected to be to everyone's advantage, and attached to positions and offices open to all (the *difference principle*).[3] For Rawls, the liberty principle governing political rights is more important, and precedes the difference principle, which governs primary goods (distributive rights), including health services.

Rawls reasons that hypothetical rational and self-interested persons in the original position will reject utilitarianism and select instead the concepts of right and justice as precedent to the good. Rawls concludes that rational self-interest dictates that one will act to protect the least well off, since anyone could be part of that group. This is termed *maximizing the minimum position (maximin)*.

When applied to primary goods, one of which is health services, Rawlsian moral theory requires egalitarianism. Egalitarianism is interpreted to mean that rational self-interested persons may limit the health services available to those in some categories, such as certain diseases or age groups, or limit services provided in certain situations. It is also rational and self-interested for persons in the original position not to make every good or service available to everyone at all times.

Rawls's theory permits the disproportionate distribution of primary goods to certain groups, but only if doing so benefits those in society who are least advantaged. This is known as the difference principle. It justifies elite social and economic status for persons such as physicians and managers if their efforts ultimately benefit the least advantaged members of society.

LINKING THEORIES AND ACTIONS

Ethical theories are developed from philosophies that are abstract and general. Rules are derived from principles. The specific judgments and actions to be applied are the final result. Beauchamp and Childress have developed a useful graphic presentation of the relationship between ethical theories (moral philosophies) and actions implementing decisions (Figure 3).

Ethical theories do not necessarily conflict with one another. Diverse philosophies may reach the same conclusion, albeit through different reasoning, by various constructs, or by applying divergent principles (e.g., the focus on ends by the utilitarian versus the focus on duty for the Kantian). The principles discussed here are critical; they should be reflected in the organization's philosophy and the personal ethic of health services managers.

Linking ethical theories and derivative principles permits development of usable guidelines. To aid that process, this discussion identifies four basic principles that provide a context for managing in the health services field. They are: 1) *respect for persons,* 2) *beneficence,* 3) *nonmaleficence,* and 4) *justice.* Sometimes utility is treated as a distinct principle, but that is somewhat artificial and potentially confusing. Here, utility is included as an adjunct to the principle of beneficence.

The theories discussed earlier support the conclusion that respect for persons is an important ethical principle. It has four elements. The first, *autonomy,* requires that one act toward others in a way that allows them to govern themselves —to choose and pursue courses of action. To do so, a person must be rational and uncoerced. Sometimes patients are or become nonautonomous (e.g., physically or mentally incapacitated patients). They are nonetheless owed respect, even though special means are required to deal with them. Autonomy underlies obtaining consent for treatment, as well as the general way an organization views and interacts with patients and staff.

Autonomy is in dynamic tension with paternalism, the concept that someone else knows what is best for another. Paternalism is a long-established tradi-

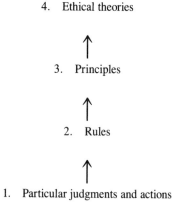

Figure 3. Hierarchy of relationships. (From Beauchamp, T.L., & Childress, J.F. [1989]. *Principles of biomedical ethics* [3rd ed.], p. 6. New York: Oxford University Press. Reprinted by permission.)

tion in health services. The earliest evidence of it is found in the Hippocratic Oath, which directs physicians to act in what they believe to be the patient's best interests. Stressing autonomy does not eliminate paternalism, but paternalism should be limited to certain situations.

The second element of respect for persons is *truth telling*. Generally, truth telling requires managers to be honest in all activities. Depending on how absolute a position is taken, this would eliminate white lies, even if they are told because it is correctly believed that if someone knew the truth harm would be caused. The morality of always telling the truth to patients is more problematic, however, depending on the circumstances. Some patients would suffer mentally and physically if told the truth about their illnesses. If so, physicians would not meet their obligation of *primum non nocere* (first, do no harm). The modern expression of this concept is nonmaleficence, discussed later in this section.

Confidentiality is the third element of the principle of respect for persons. It requires managers, as well as clinicians, to keep what they learn about patients confidential. For managers, this duty goes beyond patients. It applies to information about staff, the organization, and the community that becomes known to them in the course of their work. Exceptions to confidentiality are sometimes made because of legal requirements to report certain diseases and conditions.

The fourth element of respect is *fidelity:* doing one's duty, keeping one's word. Sometimes this is called promise keeping. We treat persons with respect when we do what we are expected to do, or what we have promised to do. Fidelity allows managers to meet the principle of respect for persons. Here, too, exceptions may be made, but they cannot be made lightly. Breaking a promise must be justified on moral grounds; it must never be done merely for convenience or self-interest.

Like respect for persons, the principle of *beneficence* is supported by the moral philosophies described earlier, although utilitarians would require it to meet the consequences test they apply. Beneficence is rooted in Hippocratic tradition, as well as in the long history of the caring professions. Beneficence may be defined as acting with charity and kindness. Applied as a principle in health services, it has a similar, but broader definition. Beneficence is a positive duty, as distinct from the principle of *nonmaleficence*, which requires refraining from actions that aggravate a problem or cause other negative results. Beneficence and nonmaleficence may be viewed as opposite ends of a continuum.

Beauchamp and Childress divide beneficence into providing benefits and balancing benefits and harms (utility).[4] Conferring benefits is firmly established in medical tradition, and failure to provide them when in a position to do so violates the concept of the duties of both clinician and manager. Balancing benefits against harms provides a philosophical basis for cost–benefit analysis, as well as other considerations of risks balanced against benefits. In this sense, it is like the principle of utility espoused by the utilitarians. Here, however, utility is only one of several considerations, and has more limited application.

The positive duty suggested by the principle of beneficence requires organizations and managers to do all they can to aid patients. There is a lesser duty to aid persons who are potential, rather than actual, patients. This distinction and its importance varies with the philosophy and mission of the organization, and whether it serves a defined population. Thus, under a principle of beneficence, the hospital operating an emergency department has no duty to scour the neighborhoods for persons in need of its assistance. When they become its patients, this relationship changes.

The second aspect of beneficence is balancing benefits and harms that could result from certain actions. This is a natural consequence of a positive duty to act in the patient's best interests. Beyond providing benefits in a positive fashion, one cannot act with kindness and charity when risks outweigh benefits. However it is interpreted, utility cannot be used to justify overriding the interests of individual patients and sacrificing them to the greater good.

The third principle applicable to managing health services organizations is *nonmaleficence*. Like beneficence, it is supported by the ethical theories discussed earlier (it must meet the consequences test to claim utilitarianism as a basis). Nonmaleficence means *primum non nocere* (first, do no harm). This dictum to physicians is equally applicable to health services managers. Beauchamp and Childress note that although nonmaleficence gives rise to specific moral rules, neither the principle nor the derivative rules can be absolute because it is often appropriate (with the patient's consent) to cause some risk, discomfort, or even harm in order to avoid greater harm or to prevent worse situations from occurring.[5] Beauchamp and Childress include the natural law concepts of extraordinary and ordinary care and double effect in the principle of nonmaleficence. These principles are considered later in this chapter. Nonmaleficence also leads managers and clinicians to avoid risks, unless potential results justify them.

The fourth principle, *justice,* is especially important for certain administrative (and clinical) decision making, such as resource allocation. It also applies to other areas of management, such as personnel policies. What is just and how does one know when justice has been achieved? Although all moral philosophies recognize the need to achieve justice, various philosophies define justice differently. Rawls defines justice as fairness. Part of that definition is that persons get what is due them. But how are fairness and just deserts defined? Aristotle's concept of justice, which is reflected in natural law, is that equals are treated equally, unequals unequally. This concept of equity is commonly used in policy analysis. Equal treatment of equals is reflected in liberty rights (e.g., universal freedom of speech). Unequal treatment of unequal persons is often used to justify a progressive income tax and redistribution of wealth: those with more income should pay a higher rate of taxes. This concept is expressed in health services delivery by expending greater resources on those who are sicker, and, thus, in need of more services.

These concepts of justice are helpful, but they do not solve the problems of definition and opinion, which are always troublesome. Macro- and microallocation of resources have received extensive consideration in the literature, but as yet there is little agreement as to operational definitions. Each organization must determine for itself how resources will be allocated. A critical criterion as to whether organizations and their clinicians and managers are acting justly is that they consistently apply clear criteria in decision processes.

MORAL PHILOSOPHY AS A BASIS FOR A PERSONAL ETHIC

This discussion of moral philosophies and derivative principles provides a framework for developing a personal ethic and subsequently analyzing ethical problems. Like philosophers, individual managers are unlikely to agree completely with all elements of a particular moral philosophy and adopt it as their own. Most managers are eclectic as they develop and reconsider a personal ethic. In general, however, the principles described here are essential to developing and maintaining appropriate relationships among patients, managers, and organizations, and should be acceptable to health services managers and the organizations they manage. It should be stressed that the four derivative principles may appropriately carry different weights, depending on the ethical issue being considered. The principle of justice requires, however, that there be a consistent ordering and weighting when the same types of ethical problems are considered.

APPLYING THE PRINCIPLES

How do the preceding principles and underlying moral philosophies assist in solving ethical problems in cases such as that of Baby Boy Doe? The principle of respect for persons implies certain duties, including autonomy. Nonautonomous persons, however, must have decisions made for them. The parents of Baby Boy Doe needed to make decisions on behalf of their son. Surrogates cannot exercise unlimited authority, however, especially when it is uncertain that a decision is in the patient's best interests. If the infant's and parents' interests differ, caregivers (including managers) have a duty under the principles of beneficence and nonmaleficence to try to persuade parents to take another course of action. This should have been attempted for Baby Boy Doe.

Extending the principles of beneficence and nonmaleficence, it is acceptable for the organization to seek legal intervention and obtain permission to treat an infant against the parents' wishes. The moral compulsion to do so is especially great when the parents do not seem to be acting in the child's best interests. But this moral duty should be exercised only as a last step. Courts intervene under a theory of *parens patriae* to permit a hospital or social welfare agency to stand *in loco parentis*. Courts always take this step reluctantly because of the common law tradition that gives parents control over reproductive and family matters, including decisions about infant children. The state is more likely to intrude as the infant reaches early childhood. As noted earlier, although it is an element of beneficence, utility is not an overriding concept that permits trampling on the rights of the person, as happened in the case of Baby Boy Doe.

Intervening has limits. Proceeding against the parents' wishes *and* without a court order is inappropriate because it breaks the law. If those caring for the infant cannot continue to do so because of their personal ethic, they should be permitted to withdraw. This option to remove oneself from a situation that is ethically intolerable should be reflected in the organization's philosophy and policies.

In applying the principle of nonmaleficence, one must consider whether it would have been less cruel to have shortened the infant's life through active euthanasia. This raises the question of whether there is a moral difference between killing and letting die. Some argue that they are morally indistinguishable because the result is the same. The analysis cannot end there, however, because it ignores critical dimensions of medical decision making.

When caregivers apply the principle of nonmaleficence they refrain from doing harm. This includes minimizing pain and suffering. Asking caregivers dedicated to preserving life to end it will cause significant role conflict. Furthermore, physicians and nurses in such roles are on a slippery slope that may lead to increasing numbers of exceptions and frequent use of positive acts to shorten lives that are deemed (by someone) not worth living.

The concept of extraordinary care is a part of the principle of nonmaleficence that developed from natural law. Ordinary care is treatment that is provided without excessive expense, pain, or inconvenience, and that offers reasonable hope of benefit. Care is considered extraordinary if it is available only in conjunction with excessive expense, pain, or other inconvenience, or if it does not offer any reasonable hope of benefit.[6] With no reasonable hope of benefit, *any* expense, pain, or inconvenience is excessive. Beauchamp and Childress conclude that the point of the distinction and its application "turn on a balance between benefits and burdens, including immediate detriment, inconvenience, and risk of harm and other costs."[7] For Baby Boy Doe, there was hope of benefit, even though correcting the atresia would have left the underlying mental retardation unaffected. Surgery would have given Baby Boy Doe a normal life for someone with his disability. That benefit justifies the use of treatment involving significant expense, pain, and/or inconvenience.

Justice is the final principle to be applied, a principle that was noted earlier to have rather divergent definitions. Rawls defines justice as fairness. Applied to the Baby Boy Doe case, one could conclude that the result was just. Fairness is arguably compatible with an enlightened self-interest expressed by persons in the original position under a veil of ignorance—a Rawlsian philosophical construct. Rational persons could decide that no life is preferable to one of significantly diminished quality, even though this seriously limits the liberty principle, which Rawls considers ultimately important.

For a Kantian, the outcome in the Baby Boy Doe case is abhorrent, because the infant is being used as a means, rather than an end. Rule utilitarians, on the other hand, would find the result acceptable. Other definitions of justice produce different conclusions. For example, if justice is defined as getting one's just deserts, it is clear that Baby Boy Doe fared badly. Applying an even cruder standard—that those equally situated should be treated equally—it is clear that had a similar problem afflicted an adult, the necessary treatment would have been rendered. For Baby Boy Doe, then, the results of applying the principle of justice are uncertain.

The final regulations about infant care published by the U.S. Department of Health and Human Services (HHS) in April, 1985, focus on beneficence and nonmaleficence. In implementing the Child Abuse Amendments of 1984 ([P.L. 98-457] amending the Child Abuse Prevention and Treatment Act of 1974), HHS gave no weight to the parents' traditional right to judge what should be done for impaired infants with life-threatening conditions. The potential problem caused by parents who may not fully understand the implications of the diagnosis and the effects of their decision is obviated by the regulations, since medical criteria applied by a knowledgeable, reasonable physician are used. Quality of life criteria cannot be considered. The preliminary regulations to implement the law made specific reference to a case such as that of Baby Boy Doe, and stated that appropriate medical treatment had to be rendered. The final regulations contain no examples, however. Nonetheless, it is apparent that HHS will view narrowly any decisions to forego treatment of impaired infants with life-threatening conditions. The regulations are discussed in Chapter 10.

As with most official efforts to regulate ethical decision making, these regulations are likely to be modified in the future. From an ethical standpoint, it is more important to bear in mind the moral considerations that should underlie public policy than to be preoccupied with the semantics of a particular enactment.

MANAGEMENT IMPLICATIONS

What are the implications of issues like these for health services managers? Such events put a heavy burden on caregivers. Whatever the decision, cases such as the case of Baby Boy Doe split the staff between those who approve and those who do not. The resulting controversy diminishes staff morale. In addi-

tion, criticism may be leveled against the management, governance, and medical staff by those who question the morality of the decision and the organization's role in it. In extreme cases, legal action may ensue.

It is crucial that the health services organization have a view (a philosophy) about matters such as these, and that it is reflected in its policies and procedures. This means the organization has explicitly formulated a course of action—a plan—it will take when confronted with such problems. This permits a deliberate response, rather than one that is reactive; inadequately considered; or governed by, rather than governing, events. At the very least, the organization must consider such issues prospectively and within the constraints of its organization philosophy.

Paradoxically, in the case of Baby Boy Doe, prior to the 1984 Child Abuse Amendments, the organization could legally do what the parents could not. Had the parents taken the infant home and allowed it to starve and dehydrate until it died, they could have been charged with child neglect or some degree of homicide or manslaughter. The organization, however, did not face the same liability. In fact, had it proceeded to repair the atresia surgically without parental consent, it would have committed battery on the infant for which it could have been sued for civil damages and the staff charged criminally. While the latter is unlikely, the hospital is legally compelled to obtain consent from the parents or legal guardian for a minor when there is no emergency.

CONCLUSION

This chapter provides information that can help the manager to develop a personal ethic and stimulate the organization to formulate a philosophy. Few managers will disagree as to the importance of the principles of respect for persons, beneficence, nonmaleficence, and justice. However, not all managers will unequivocally embrace the principles and underlying moral philosophies discussed here, and they may not agree as to their weighting or priority. Chapter 2 suggests a methodology that managers can use in solving ethical problems.

NOTES

1. Robert Hunt and John Arras, eds., *Issues in Modern Medicine,* 2nd ed. (Palo Alto, CA: Mayfield Publishing Co., 1983), 27.

2. Edgar Bodenheimer, *Jurisprudence: The Philosophy and Method of the Law,* rev. ed. (Cambridge: Harvard University Press, 1974), 23–24.

3. John Rawls, *A Theory of Justice* (Cambridge: Belknap Press, 1971), 60.

4. Tom L. Beauchamp and James F. Childress, *Principles of Biomedical Ethics,* 3rd ed. (New York: Oxford University Press, 1989), 195.

5. Ibid., 122.

6. Gerald Kelly, "The Duty to Preserve Life," *Theological Studies* (December 12, 1951): 550.

7. Beauchamp and Childress, *Biomedical Ethics,* 153.

2

∞

RESOLVING ETHICAL ISSUES

Mᴀɴᴀɢᴇʀs ᴀʀᴇ ᴘʀᴏʙʟᴇᴍ sᴏʟᴠᴇʀs. It is the reason they are hired—organizations without problems do not need managers. Some problems burst on the scene. There is no doubt something is amiss when a wildcat strike occurs among the nursing staff, or when the local newspaper attacks the organization. Other problems are hard to uncover, and often give no clear evidence or warning. They must be identified and treated early, because undetected, they will grow, and may threaten the organization's survival. Solving them is similar to detecting cancer and providing early treatment. In the words of the old adage, "a stitch in time saves nine."

Successful managers have highly developed conceptual and problem identification skills. Preventing or at least identifying and solving ethical problems with minimal organization disruption is as critical as solving management problems that primarily affect personnel or finance. It is almost certain, too, that ethical problems will have implications for traditional management areas, and that traditional management problems will have ethical dimensions. It is important in this comparison to note that techniques and skills employed in solving ethical problems are essentially the same as those needed to solve the traditional type of management problem. Problem solving is a generic process that applies to both types of problems.

PRESENCE OF ETHICAL PROBLEMS

Many managers believe they are inadequately prepared to recognize ethical problems, and that they are even less able to solve such problems. This belief underestimates the value of the typical managers' credentials. Identifying ethical problems is primarily a matter of mindset, attitude, and applying common sense when reviewing or analyzing a situation. Determining the ethical dimensions of a problem is usually less difficult than developing alternatives for their solution and implementing the solution selected. Developing and implementing solutions are more likely to require assistance from within the organization, or even from outside.

Managers who see their role primarily as solving problems of staffing, directing, budgeting, controlling, organizing, coordinating, integrating, and planning are more in need of sensitivity to ethical issues than postgraduate education in philosophy. Methodologies similar to those used to solve traditional management problems can be used to solve ethical problems, whether administrative or biomedical. That generic process is discussed later in this chapter. However, traditional management issues often overshadow, and may even overwhelm, ethical dimensions. In addition, ethical aspects can be subtle, thus making initial identification and efforts toward solution more difficult.

With authority delegated by the governing body, managers represent the organization. The organization's philosophy provides a general context for the manager's activities and decision making, as discussed in Chapter 3. But the presence of an organizational philosophy does not eliminate the manager's need for a personal ethic. The personal ethic provides individual managers with a framework for action, and permits greater refinement of principles, rules, and particular judgments and actions than is likely to be present in the statement of philosophy developed by the typical health services organization. It bears repeating that each human being is a moral agent whose actions have moral consequences. Conduct cannot be excused because someone claims to have been following orders. This is true whether the orders emanate from the governing body or from elsewhere. Orders from lawfully constituted authorities, such as courts, pose a special problem. Moral agents who consider such orders unjust may decide to engage in acts of civil disobedience, but in doing so they must be prepared to bear societally imposed sanctions. The ethical (moral) implications of acts must be considered independently.

Occasionally, there may be a conflict between the organization's ethic, as expressed in its philosophy, and the manager's personal ethic. Since the organization is a bureaucracy that often behaves as though it had a life of its own, it is incumbent on the manager to think through carefully the implications of acquiescing to the organization's policy. This follows from the concept of moral agency. It often seems easier to go along in order to get along than to risk one's position by speaking out. The dilemma for those considering professional dissent or those who may become whistleblowers is one that seems to confront too few managers. Managers must recognize both the distinction between and the integration of an organizational and a personal ethic. They must not go about their daily tasks with little thought about the ethical context of their work.

In terms of the problem-solving methodology described later in the chapter, the organization's philosophy and the individual's personal ethic are vital. They provide the framework and context within which the manager functions. They enhance sensitization to and identification and solution of ethical problems so that managers can approach such problems as they approach traditional management problems.

ADMINISTRATIVE ETHICAL ISSUES

Leadership is an essential part of management. It includes setting goals, establishing direction, and guiding the organization. These activities are more ethics sensitive than are the more routine managerial activities. Day-to-day activities often seem value free, but even they are based on earlier actions rooted in ethical principles, whether or not those principles are identified and expressly stated. However management functions are interpreted, human beings cannot escape their role as moral agents. Managers set a tone and establish a context for the organization and its staff, especially when they function as leaders. They cannot avoid scrutiny of evidence of their personal ethic, as well as its congruence with the organization's philosophy.

Managers hold positions of trust. These positions may not be used for personal advantage or aggrandizement, and managers must not act in any way that carries the slightest hint of wrongdoing. These are essential elements of a personal ethic if one seeks to be an effective leader. Actions should be judged by applying the ethical principles developed in Chapter 1. An additional effective way of clarifying the pragmatic effect of an action is to step back and view what is being done or contemplated as though one were an outsider. How do the public and colleagues see it? This "seen through the eyes of others" or "light of public scrutiny" standard for judging action is very helpful. Using a cynic's standard is not useful. Meeting it is impossible, because cynics find problems even when it is unreasonable to do so. Skepticism is, however, a useful criterion for managers to apply as they seek to understand how their actions might be seen. A criterion that should never be used is the criterion of being discovered—an "if you don't get caught, it's okay" standard. Such a standard negates the need for codes of ethics and substitutes a criterion that encourages deviousness.

In a way quite different from that of a personal ethic or an organization's philosophy, the law provides a baseline of what is considered ethical. As noted in the Introduction, comparisons with the law are useful. They guide us only partially, however, because the law is a minimum standard of conduct, and no manager can effectively lead by meeting minimum requirements. The manager *qua* leader must set an example that substantially surpasses the standard expected of others. Professional codes of ethics also guide conduct and provide frames of reference. They require a higher, more demanding level of performance than the law, but they, too, should not be viewed as incorporating all expectations of ethical performance.

Is it reasonable to argue that where one stands on administrative ethics depends on where one sits? Does the concept of "rank hath its privileges" apply to managing health services? Some senior managers act in a fashion that suggests that they believe it does. It is easy to find situations in which subordinates are reprimanded for behavior that goes unpunished at the upper echelons. In these cases, it is a matter of "do as I say, not as I do"; or "what is sauce for the goose is not sauce for the gander." These managers apply a double standard. Few persons can fail to distinguish words from actions; applying a double standard gives staff a clear message of cynicism and inconsistency. Consequently, a manager's ability to lead is diminished.

Managers can become aware and sensitive about ethical issues in several ways. They should be avid readers of both the popular press and professional literature. Professional codes of ethics are valuable for guiding and understanding the parameters of acceptable actions. Not to be forgotten is intuition and hunch—that sixth sense that says something is wrong. It can be cultivated and nurtured to alert the manager to the presence of an ethical problem.

Identifying ethical problems of all types means focusing on the principles of respect for persons, beneficence, nonmaleficence, and justice; asking if the actions contemplated violate them; and determining whether such a violation is justified by special circumstances. A questioning mind permits the manager to consider the situation further or seek assistance, as appropriate. Indentifying administrative ethical problems requires attention to detail and constant vigilance.

BIOMEDICAL ETHICAL ISSUES

All actual and contemplated interactions with patients represent potential sources of ethical problems. These problems range from paternalism to consent, from truth telling to the right to die. Managers may feel uncomfortable and out of place trying to solve biomedical ethical problems. They should not. *Medicine and the clinician provide key information that assists in making informed ethical decisions, but the decision itself is ethical (moral), not clinical.* This distinction between the clinical and ethical aspects of biomedical decision making is critical, and must not be forgotten by managers. Managers will gain confidence as they have greater experience and exposure. Their participation is needed not only because greater medical staff/administration interaction results in a more effective and efficient organization, but because all biomedical problems have administrative dimensions. In this regard, the manager's involvement is critical.

The manager does not supersede the clinician, but the manager has an important role in preventing or solving biomedical ethical problems. Examples include serving on institutional ethics committees (IECs) and institutional review boards (IRBs) and determining resource allocation. These are discussed in later chapters. In addition, managers are major actors in developing and putting into practice the policies, procedures, and rules that implement the organization's philosophy.

As noted earlier, managers need not take postgraduate courses in philosophy or bioethics to identify the presence of potential problems (although such courses might be helpful). Primarily, learning to identify potential ethical problems requires sensitization, an inquiring mind, and a reasonably well developed personal ethic. Questions such as "Is the patient being treated as I would wish to be?", "Is the patient protected from unnecessary harm?", and "Does the consent process adequately inform the patient about what is being done?" are useful in identifying bioethical problems. As with all problem solving, asking the right questions may be the most important part of the process.

An important role for managers is stimulating the medical staff and other caregivers to develop the necessary expertise to prevent or deal effectively with biomedical ethical problems. To do so, caregivers must have procedures and rules to follow. Here, the manager's role as a catalyst is the same as that played in traditional administrative activities. Regrettably, the codes of administrative ethics provide little guidance in addressing biomedical ethical issues.

PROBLEM SOLVING

Unresolved ethical problems will have the same destructive effect on an organization as problems involving personnel, finance, or the medical staff. Therefore, it is imperative that managers have a methodology for solving them. This poses some difficulties, however, since few managers have formal training in ethics. Ethical issues may seem more subtle than management problems, and since managers tend to be pragmatic, they are not inclined to grapple with apparent nuances. Sometimes ethical problems are combined with issues that appear to overshadow the ethical dimensions. Furthermore, managers may consider ethical issues less important than other issues, perhaps because they do not comprehend their potentially devastating effect. These obstacles can be overcome, however.

In 1910, John Dewey, the American educator and philosopher, wrote in his book *How We Think* that there are three stages of problem solving: 1) identifying the problem, 2) identifying the alternatives, and 3) determining which alternative is best. Successful managers implicitly or explicitly use a similar process. They include: identifying the problem in terms of both the current manifestation (which may be only a symptom) and the underlying cause; developing alternative solutions and the decision criteria by which to judge them acceptable, unacceptable, or optimum; preparing an implementation plan for the solution that is selected; and developing a means of evaluating the solution once it has been implemented.

Philosophers employ a similar methodology to analyze ethical problems. They call it moral reasoning, and its components are surprisingly similar to the manager's problem-solving methodology.

Analyzing—separating the overall structure of a problem in a particular case into its major components;

Weighing—assessing strengths and weaknesses of various alternatives which could be used in solving the problem by balancing them against one another;

Justifying—providing a compelling and sufficient moral reason that appeals to an established moral principle, such as "Always tell the truth." (Any such principle must be compatible with the organization's philosophy *and* the manager's personal ethic.);

Choosing—selecting one or more of the available alternatives, preferably on the basis of a position that can be and has been shown to be justified;

Evaluating—reexamining the choices and their justifications, identifying unanswered questions, and relating decisions about one particular case to similar cases.[1]

Problem solving can be divided into two basic types:

> The specific focus on problem solving is rooted in two broad models, the rational and the heuristic. Problem definition is addressed differently by each of these models. The rational model (sometimes identified with programmed decisions) assumes that one is faced with a specific problem and focuses primarily on a search for the optimal solution.
>
> Operations research, for example, is primarily a quantitative expression of this approach applied to a wide range of management issues. In the hospital, it includes problems such as work scheduling, e.g., developing a computer program that maximizes the preferred work schedule of a large number of nurses, or a PERT chart used to schedule the construction of a new building. These and similar problem-solving techniques are important for an organization, and help it to establish patterns for problem solving.
>
> The heuristic model (sometimes identifed with nonprogrammed decisions, or a learning model) acknowledges that some problems may be more diffusely defined, poorly structured, and are often not routine. It focuses upon an iterative process of dealing with problem definition, as well as solution. Heuristic general problem-solving techniques have been suggested for training administrators. Heuristic problem-solving approaches which are quantitative and computer-based have been advocated.[2]

This distinction between rational and heuristic models suggests that solving ethical problems requires heuristic techniques. First, however, process components must be separated from substance components, and ethical problems that recur and have similar features must be distinguished from problems that are unique and unlikely to be repeated. Process components are more amenable to analysis and solution by the rational model than are substance components. Those that recur and have similar features are also more likely to be solved using the rational model. But even here, efforts to implement the process may uncover unique or subtle problems of substance, such as the relative authority of different persons in the decision process. The two problem-solving theories are not mutually exclusive, however, and the heuristic model can often benefit from using a rational model for portions of the analysis. Thus, problem solvers should not choose one model to the exclusion of the other.

Master's degree programs in health services administration, as well as master of business administration programs, typically cover problem-solving methodologies. These methodologies are also useful in solving ethical problems, and are similar to the generic problem-solving model presented in Figure 4. That model is shown as two-dimensional, but it should be conceptualized with a third dimension, time. In this respect, it is like a cork screw: while the problem-solving process cycles from the point of problem analysis to evaluation of actual results, the whole process moves through time.

In Figure 4, problem analysis begins when the manager objectively or intuitively finds something amiss. In typical problem solving for management problems, it is here that actual results deviate from desired or expected results, or a situation develops requiring an organizational response. Examples of man-

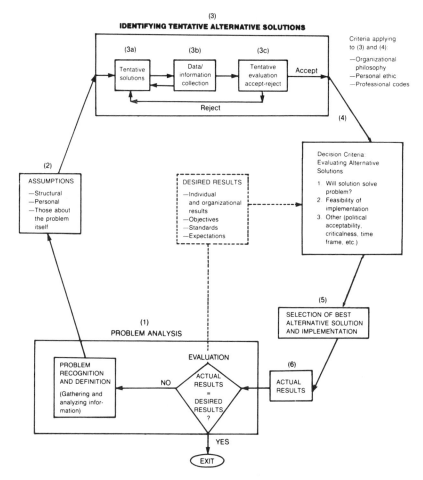

Figure 4.   Schema for solving ethical problems. (Adapted from Rakich, J.S., Longest, B.B., Jr., & Darr, K. [1985]. *Managing health services organizations* [2nd ed.], p. 247. Philadelphia: W.B. Saunders.)

agement situations needing attention are: a declining or rapidly increasing admission rate in the outpatient department, increased turnover among staff in a department, more uneaten food returned from patient rooms (or the cafeteria) to the dietary department, or an announcement that a competing emergicenter is opening or an existing one is closing. Some of these potential problems are foreseen through analysis of routinely collected data; others emerge only when the event occurs. The more apparent the problem, the more likely it is that the rational rather than the heuristic model can be used.

Similarly, the ethical dimensions of some situations are often apparent. If a patient is diagnosed as being in a persistent vegetative state (PVS), an ethical problem with both clinical and administrative dimensions exists. Similarly, an ethical problem is present when the organization lacks an effective consent process. Such situations have little need for a heuristic problem-solving process.

For either type of problem, however, these are only potential problems until management defines a situation as a problem that must be solved. Sometimes, before any deliberate resolution of the situation's ethical dimensions occurs, events cause the problem to disappear (e.g., the patient in a persistent vegetative state has a cardiac arrest and cannot be resuscitated). Although the problem has disappeared, it has not been resolved by solving the problem.

Berry and Seavey argue that problem definitions "are fundamentally subjective (and) . . . are not objective, concrete realities; they are perceptions of reality."[3] This statement is correct insofar as it bears on perceptions of cause and effect, but it requires qualification when applied in certain situations. For example, striking housekeeping workers walking a picket line represent a verifiable fact, and will be defined as a problem needing solution by any manager. Perceptions (subjectivity) vary in determining cause, or in identifying the underlying situation (problem) that may be the cause. Views of problems and their solution are affected by the positions held and responsibilities of the persons involved. Certainly, the housekeeping workers have a different explanation of the strike's causes than does management.

In solving problems that are primarily ethical, context is much more important than it is in dealing with management problems with few ethical dimensions. The context of an ethical problem is the philosophy and mission of the organization applied by a manager who has a personal ethic and is a moral agent. Once a situation with ethical dimensions has been recognized and defined as a problem, it must be understood. This necessitates gathering and analyzing information about its extent and character, which may be available through existing data systems or may require special efforts. Managers solving ethical problems are likely to experience the same deficiencies of data that they confront when considering other types of problems.

In box (2) in Figure 4, managers make assumptions about the problem, personal implications and views, and structure within which the problem arises. In the case of Baby Boy Doe, staff were undoubtedly affected. It is reasonable to assume that in such a case, staff will become depressed and angry and morale will decline. It may also be assumed that few staff will be so upset that they will resign, turn to a union, or refuse to work in the nursery. Assumptions such as these require judgment by managers, and could result in a decision to ignore the situation (i.e., not define it as a problem requiring solution). Such a result depends largely on the organizational philosophy and the individual manager's personal ethic. Choosing to do nothing is always an option, if it meets the decision criteria, and this may be the best alternative in many situations. It must, however, never be the choice by default.

Identifying and assessing possible alternative solutions, shown in box (3), is the preliminary review of options. Here, decision makers brainstorm to identify creative solutions. It is imperative that managers solving ethical problems, whether administrative or biomedical, be mindful of the organization's philosophy, as well as their personal ethic. Unless changing those constraints is possible, solutions falling outside them must be discarded. To ignore or apply these constraints arbitrarily creates inconsistencies and discontinuities that eventually cause major problems for the organization and for the manager. Other general criteria are also applied here.

If alternative solutions pass this preliminary screening, they are subjected to a detailed assessment. This necessitates comparing each option against specific decision criteria. As shown in box (4) of Figure 4, these criteria include: the time needed to solve the problem, real costs of all kinds (e.g., political, financial, reputation), opportunity costs, feasibility of implementation, adequacy of solving the problem, and benefits derived. Applying more specific criteria results in better solutions and outcomes. A major benefit of greater specificity in the process is that it requires managers to review, analyze, and in other ways become as precise as possible, not only in defining the problem, but in considering and selecting the alternative that best solves it. This is a useful exercise because it hones management decision making. Some managers may go a step farther and weight, or assign relative values to, decision criteria, since some are likely to be more important than others.

Prior to and after selecting the alternative, the manager must deal with implementation and evaluation. A common failing among managers is that they put great effort into developing a solution and beginning implementation, and then turn to other matters. The result is that the solution flounders even before it is fully implemented. Implementing the solution should receive as much attention as selecting it. A means of evaluation must be included in each solution so that difficulties can be identified and corrective action taken in a timely manner. These corrective actions are a subset of the problem-solving process, and may involve the same or similar steps.

This problem-solving methodology is useful whether decision making addresses ethical problems solved by a single manager, by management, by governing body committees, or by specially established committees, such as institutional ethics committees (IECs), infant care review committees (ICRCs), or institutional review boards (IRBs). It is useful whether directed at solving one problem, considering guidelines to address a class of problems, or developing a process used later to bring a similar methodology to bear on solving individual problems or groups of problems. Regardless of the source of decision making, once the process is established and policies (which have gone through a similar problem-solving methodology) have been formulated and implemented, operating procedures and rules will be established. That means an issue (e.g., consent) has been considered, and the ethically acceptable policies, procedures, and processes have been identified. Therefore, as a general rule, the majority of ethical problems will be prevented. Exceptions and special attention will be necessary when the facts differ sufficiently from the assumptions implicit in the policy and the procedures derived from it.

In this regard, it is unnecessary to distinguish administrative from biomedical ethical issues. In terms of general policies and guidelines, both types of problems should be considered prospectively. Resulting policies and procedures will cover the majority of predictable, recurring ethical problems. That is why, for example, a governing body adopts a conflict of interest policy applicable to itself and management staff. Despite the usefulness of general guidelines and specific rules, however, problems do arise, especially as to their interpretation and application. It bears repeating that the problem-solving model discussed earlier is usable at two levels: general policy development and consideration of individual cases.

Although in most ways implementing solutions to administrative or biomedical ethical problems is the same as it is for management problems, some distinctions should be noted. Ethical issues often involve a high level of emotion. Examples are situations that suggest a manager has behaved unethically (administrative ethics), or that a patient's view of life and death has been violated or challenged (biomedical ethics). This requires that the manager and staff who work to solve such problems have a much greater sensitivity to human factors, and that they understand that they are not dealing with units of production or ordinary services. Another distinction is that both administrative and biomedical ethical issues often have significant legal consequences. These are especially important in biomedical ethical problems. Even though all health services organizations should apply a standard much higher than the minimum set by the law, mistakes do occur, and occasionally there are problems that bring in lawyers. A third distinction is that there may be negative public relations consequences both inside and outside the organization.

DEVELOPING A PERSONAL ETHIC

Health services managers enter the field as adults who have already developed at least an implicit personal ethic. In developing that ethic, managers have been affected by a host of influences, including family and friends, religious principles and teachings, secular education, and the law. It is in this context that adults become managers, and in which a personal ethic about management is developed. For many, their ethic may be only an intuitive sense of right and wrong, with no clearly identifiable source or explicitly defined code of conduct.

Developing a personal ethic necessitates being introspective, asking "Who am I?", "How do I view certain actions or activities?", "What do I consider unethical?", "What is morally right or wrong?" This knowledge of self furthers an understanding of others as well. Such understanding is critically important as managers search for the "right" answer to ethical problems. Both new and experienced health services managers draw on a number of sources in developing and refining their personal ethics. Chief among them are the codes of ethics of professional associations, educational socialization, and the association and pressure of peers, subordinates, and superiors.

In selecting the principles that will be included in a personal ethic, managers should apply the criteria of comprehensiveness, consistency, and coherence. Do the principles apply to the broadest possible range of ethical issues? How useful and applicable are they in solving ethical problems? Do they use the scientific method in terms of exactness, systemization, and predictability? Are the ethical conceptions clear and consistent? Are they in conflict with or consistent with other knowledge or life experiences? Are they reasonably adaptable to a changing world? Even though the criteria of comprehensiveness, consistency, and coherence are not applied with the rigor of a moral philosopher, they should be kept in mind when judging, developing, or reconsidering a personal ethic, as well as when analyzing the ethics of others or disputing their reasoning or conclusions.

In addition to the manager's personal ethic, the organization's philosophy is vital to ethical decision making. It is tempting to say that the personal ethic is and ought to remain the most important. One cannot, however, ignore the realities of bureaucratic life. Some sectarian health services organizations require complete congruence between the personal and the organizational ethic by hiring no one above midlevel management who is not an adherent of that faith. The wisdom of such a policy is discussed later. Suffice it to say here that in modern, complex health services organizations, there exists a significant potential for discontinuity between the philosophy of the organization and that of its managers. The extent to which these philosophies must be identical, or even congruent, is unclear, however. It is likely that the organization's philosophy will be more instrumental in developing the personal ethic of a younger, less experienced manager. Like other groups, managers, too, become set in their ways.

CONCLUSION

In solving ethical problems, successful managers implicitly or explicitly use a problem-solving methodology similar to that shown in Figure 4. Effectively solving ethical issues requires the same attention. Managers cannot ignore ethical problems, and they must effectively participate in solving them. This does not mean that health services managers supersede physicians or other clinical staff where biomedical ethics are involved. It does mean that in an effort to operationalize the principles developed earlier, managers must participate effectively in solving ethical problems. By the nature of the job, the manager may serve as team leader and catalyst. Being the organization's conscience is consistent with the manager's role as moral agent in a position of ethical leadership. In terms of administrative ethics, the manager's role is indisputably preeminent.

Successful managers have a well-developed personal ethic and a clear understanding of their own views on matters of administrative and biomedical ethical issues. This ethic has been defined by drawing from a wide variety of sources. A personal ethic cannot be chiseled in stone. It evolves over time. While one's basic view of the world is likely to remain relatively stable, experience, maturation, and technological developments affect one's personal ethic.

NOTES

1. Frank Harron, John Burnside, and Tom Beauchamp, *Health and Human Values* (New Haven: Yale University Press, 1983), 4.

2. David E. Berry and John W. Seavey, "Reiteration of Problem Definition in Health Services Administration," *Hospital & Health Services Administration 29,* no. 2 (March/April 1984): 58.

3. Ibid., 59.

II

∞

GUIDELINES IN MAKING
ETHICAL DECISIONS

A SIGNIFICANT PROBLEM WITH APPLIED ETHICS, whether biomedical or administrative, is that many written and unwritten codes influence a manager's behavior. These result from family background, religious orientation and training, professional affiliations and allegiances, and a too often ill-defined personal code of moral conduct—an amalgam of intellect, experience, education, and relationships. Such codes are typically vague, perhaps even contradictory. This problem, added to a generally high level of tolerance for varying views, causes many managers to believe ethical problems have no answers, only agonizing and morally impossible choices. Often, too, events begin to control, rather than being controlled by, managers, who find themselves being shaped rather than shaping.

One attribute of many professions, including health services management, is that their members engage in activities that involve a strong element of service to humanity. A continuing problem for health services managers and the profession is determining the demarcation between private and professional lives. If the manager's private conduct breaches the profession's code of ethics, the profession may take disciplinary action.

There is the continuing dynamic and tension between the private and professional aspects of the manager's life (and the lives of most other employees) and the health services organization's philosophy and mission statement. These are the organization's basic law, and guide its policy development and implementation. An important question is, "Must the manager's philosophy be identical to the organization's?"

Chapters 3 and 4 suggest how to develop an organizational philosophy and examine its importance in providing health services. Codes of ethics and their role in guiding health services managers, as well as helping them develop personal ethics, are discussed. The dynamic between the organization's philosophy and the manager's code is analyzed.

Means by which managers and organizations can obtain assistance in solving ethical problems are considered in Chapter 5. Specialized committees whose attention focuses on various types of ethical problems and other means of obtaining assistance are suggested. As a moral agent, the manager remains the focal point of efforts to prevent or identify and solve ethical problems.

3

∞

ORGANIZATIONAL
PHILOSOPHY AND MISSION

MANAGERS CONFRONT A VARIETY of moral and symbolic issues omnipresent in health services organizations. The focus here is on moral issues that include the need for the organization to define and adopt values and principles—a philosophy—from which it derives its mission, and the means by which that mission is achieved. This exercise prospectively resolves conflicts among competing but legitimate ends. The sequence described is the theoretical ideal. It is as likely that the organization's mission is defined first, or evolves as a consequence of past action, within the context of an implicit, rather than explicit, organizational philosophy. This chapter describes the importance of identifying the moral values and principles that govern development of a mission statement, and ascertaining if they are reflected throughout the organization by the staff.

Mission is necessarily limited by, and a function of, the organization's physical location, size, resources, and other aspects of its internal and external environment. Most of these factors can be affected, but usually only over time. If any of these factors changes, it is necessary to review the organization's mission. Other elements in the mission are a direct function of the moral values and principles identified as appropriate by the organization. An acute care hospital may or may not perform abortions. The decision derives from a determination that such a service is compatible (or incompatible) with its moral values and principles, as formulated and interpreted by its governing body. An issue such as abortion raises other questions, the answers to which should be consistent with the organization's stand on abortion. For example, is performing abortions compatible with legally required efforts to provide medically indicated treatment to aborted fetuses? Some organizations avoid these questions and the attendant ethical implications by simply adhering to the law, that is, they equate legality and morality. For many situations, this only partially solves the problem, since, as will be seen, the law is very poorly developed in a number of areas in which administrative and biomedical ethical problems arise.

Just because a governing body develops and adopts a statement of philosophy reflecting certain moral values and principles is no reason to believe that the staff agrees. Personnel in organizations typically pay little attention to such matters, and the health services field is no exception. Many personnel may not even know what the philosophy is, despite reasonable efforts by the organization to communicate it. Even if they understand the philosophy, many may have no commitment to it. If staff pay little attention to what the organization has stated in terms of its moral values and principles, it is not surprising that they pay even less attention to what the organization should have said, but has not. For those employees, the organization is merely a place to work. They do their jobs, and are unconcerned about what the upper echelons establish as a context for service delivery. Short of major discontinuity—when even sabotage may occur—members of the staff rarely overtly challenge what is being done. If a challenge is made, results tend to be negative, not positive, in outcome and effect.

Consider how much more effective the organization could be if it were built on a system of shared values and goals. Of course, exceptions to policies might be needed in certain situations and for some persons. Adequately communicated to and accepted by the staff, a goal as simple as "getting the caring back into curing" could reap great rewards for the organization through improved efficiency and better patient care and relations. Having employees headed in the same direction—a direction known in advance and recognized as important elsewhere in the organization (e.g., by managers at performance appraisal time)—will positively affect attitude, productivity, and effectiveness.

ORGANIZATIONAL PHILOSOPHY

The starting point from which an organization undertakes to solve ethical problems is its philosophy. The statement of philosophy identifies moral values and principles reflecting right and wrong for the organization and, thus, distinguishes the acceptable from the unacceptable. It is helpful if such a philosophy is sufficiently precise so that performance in achieving it can be evaluated. At a minimum, of course, the statement of philosophy must be consistent with the law.

The organizational philosophy is different from the mission statement and should be developed separately. The philosophy provides a context for the mission statement; the mission statement is subordinate to it. Nonetheless, some organizations include references to values in their mission statements. A mission statement that "the corporation owns and operates hospitals to provide care for the sick and injured" provides no information about the moral context of the care. A mission statement that "the hospital provides care for the sick and injured in the context of Christian principles" is imprecise, but provides a clearer value or moral context than the first.

Anecdotal evidence suggests that most health services organizations do not have specific, expressed philosophies with measurable components. Nonetheless, a de facto or functional philosophy can be identified because the aggregate effect of decisions and actions taken by the governing body and management have implicit, albeit ill-defined, philosophical bases. Results of management actions may be contradictory or inconsistent, and this suggests another negative aspect of not prospectively determining a comprehensive philosophy. This problem is reflected in a lack of continuity that may lead to incompatible policies, procedures, and rules. The effect will be to diminish the organization's efficiency.

The theme of identified and shared values is a major thrust of the widely acclaimed book *In Search of Excellence* (Peters & Waterman, 1982). The authors quote Thomas J. Watson, Jr., former president of IBM: " . . . the basic philosophy of an organization has far more to do with its achievements than do technological or economic resources, organizational structure, innovation and timing."[1] The context of his statement is the focus on consumer service that has had such an important positive effect on IBM's reputation and financial success. This is a unique attitude in a company with many characteristics of a product industry (although IBM considers itself a service organization). If consumer and service are that important to the success of IBM, consider how much more important they are in a field such as health services delivery. These emphases are especially noteworthy as organizations in the health services system increasingly face the competitive challenges met so successfully by IBM. The centrality of shared values is shown in Figure 5, the 7-S Framework developed by the consulting firm of McKinsey and Company.

In their book *Corporate Cultures,* Deal and Kennedy identify characteristics shared by successful companies:

- They stand for something—that is, they have a clear and explicit philosophy about how they aim to conduct their business.
- Management pays a great deal of attention to shaping and fine-tuning these values to conform to the economic and business environment of the company and to communicating them to the organization.
- These values are known and shared by all the people who work for the company—from the production worker right through to the ranks of senior management.[2]

Building on this concept of the importance of shared values or philosophy, Deal and Kennedy describe the important elements of a culture: 1) shared values and beliefs about success in the environment, 2) heroes who epitomize those values and beliefs, 3) rituals that prescribe how all critical activities are to be carried out, 4) ceremonies that celebrate successes of the culture, and 5) stories and storytellers to keep the mythology of the culture alive.[3]

In a more recent discussion of corporate cultures Kennedy wrote:

Culture isn't a single thing. It's not a budget; it's not a plan; it's not the shape of a building. It is an integrated pattern of all the things that go on in an organization on a day-to-day basis. Each company has its own unique culture, values, and standards communicated internally by style, dress, expectations, and assumptions.

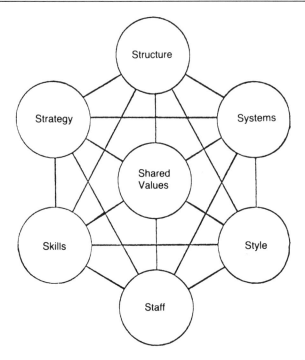

Figure 5. The McKinsey 7-S Framework. (From McKinsey & Company, Inc. Reprinted with permission).

New people in the workplace find out what is expected of them because their peers take them aside and say, "Look, don't wear jeans here. Come in to work on time, or you do this or that." They lay out some of the unwritten rules of behavior that are required for entrance into your workplace. That's how culture transmits itself to each new generation of persons. They don't come in and invent a whole new style of organization. They come in and learn from those around them what's going on in the organization and how they are expected to behave.[4]

There are barriers to establishing strong corporate cultures in any organization; they are especially present in health services organizations. Some barriers particularly relevant to hospitals include:

- Hospitals must serve diverse medical needs of heterogeneous populations;
- The number of external variables [forces outside the organization which affect it] is much greater for hospitals than in ordinary business enterprise;
- Hospital outcomes are difficult to define and to measure;
- It is difficult to nurture the keen proprietary sense of individual endeavors among leadership and management staff at all levels;
- Hospital board members are not active participants in its culture;
- Hospital physicians are a subculture, and peer acceptance and recognition, participation in professional activities, and stature based on professional contribution and expertise are more important than the rewards of belonging to a particular hospital;

- Elaborate peer reward systems in nursing are complicated by a deep search for professional identity;
- Increasingly, support staff and especially allied medical personnel tend to have a professional identification independent of the hospital; and
- Another special subculture in hospitals are the administrators who are caught between the role of facilitating the delivery of medical care, and that of running a cost-effective "business," and as a result often isolate themselves from other subcultures.[5]

Beyond these factors, and implicit in them, is the need for managers to view their relationships with patients in a consistent fashion. Paying lip service to the organization's avowed goal of patient care but in fact stressing economic or other nonpatient considerations is a contradiction that will not be lost on staff, who will respond to real, rather than platitudinous, incentives.

Management must know and understand the culture and values in its organization. As importantly, it must know how they mesh with or diverge from those the organization wishes to develop. The organization can mold a culture, but it cannot move faster than or in directions opposed or misunderstood by those in the organization. This congruence is critical. The organization's philosophy and derivative mission statement are the major reference points for its corporate culture and subordinated activities. All efforts to develop excellence are a function of them.

Closely linked to the concept of an organizational philosophy and corporate culture is management's view of the organization's personnel. For those familiar with McGregor's Theories X and Y or Maslow's need hierarchy, the theme of developing an effective corporate culture has a familiar ring. The organization's view of its employees is likely to be similar to its view of its patients. Dysfunction is rife in an organization that treats employees in an adversarial and distrustful fashion, or as a means to an end, while simultaneously urging those same employees to treat patients with dignity and respect. Employees will see the hypocrisy and respond negatively. Peters and Waterman sound this same theme as they quote Thomas J. Watson, Jr.: "IBM's philosophy is largely contained in three simple beliefs. I want to begin with what I think is the most important: our respect for the individual. This is a simple concept, but in IBM it occupies a major portion of management time."[6]

CONTENT OF A PHILOSOPHY STATEMENT

Organization

The principles enunciated in the organizational philosophy are broad; the mission statement puts flesh on the skeleton. The philosophy statement provides the context and the operative values—it gives delivery of health services a life, a meaning—and recognizes that these values are unique and represent more than just a means of delivering a product or rendering a service. The mission statement and the goals, objectives, policies, and procedures derived from the philosophy describe the organization's reason for being. One health system describes its philosophy (values) with a list of its beliefs:[7]

- human life
- wholism
- shared ministry
- peacemaking
- human dignity
- preference for the poor
- business ethics
- advocacy

One of its member hospitals has developed a mission statement based on this philosophy. It is a statement of activities that references the healing mission of the Roman Catholic church and a commitment to provide "within the limits of our resources, compassionate and quality holistic care to all in our community, within which we especially cherish the poor."[8] The beliefs of the Franciscan Health System and the mission statement of Saint Mary Hospital are reprinted in Appendix A.

Moral considerations important to the organization should be addressed in the statement of philosophy. They can include the organization's position on specific biomedical ethical issues. If, for example, its view of the sanctity of life prohibits performing abortions, this should be stated. The organization's view of its relationship with patients, staff (including those, such as physicians, who are not salaried employees), community, and other institutions should be described. It is important that the statement be written in sufficient detail that performance measures can be developed and applied.

Consistent with the moral philosophies and derivative principles discussed earlier, the organization's philosophy must emphasize the importance of ensuring respect for all persons, seeking to benefit the patient, and protecting the patient from any untoward result. It is desirable, too, that principles of justice be addressed in the philosophy. These principles are inherent in the independent relationship between the organization and the patient, and are not superseded by the relationship between the physician and the patient. Through its philosophy, the organization also implicitly or explicitly expresses its accountability to the public, regardless of whether the institution is publicly or privately owned.

Relationship to Patients

One cannot imagine a health services organization that fails to identify its role vis-à-vis patients from the standpoint of respect for persons, beneficence, nonmaleficence, and justice. These principles stress providing medical services to the patient with respect and in a manner that enhances human dignity. Staff members must know of their responsibilities and duties toward patients in this regard. Patients are the primary reason the organization exists, and all efforts are directed at meeting patient needs in delivering high-quality services safely.

Williams and Donnelly emphasize this relationship in *Medical Care Quality and the Public Trust.*[9] They argue that accountability to the patient takes precedence over any other duty of the governing body or any relationship between the governing body and any other person or entity, including the medical staff. They assert that this accountability extends so far that if medical malpractice has harmed a patient who is unaware of that harm, the hospital has a duty to inform the patient. This position is radical, and is not likely to be received positively by many health services governing bodies or managers, although they may agree with it intellectually.

There are major economic hazards to accepting and implementing such a philosophy, especially in an acute care hospital with a voluntary medical staff. The new emphasis on marketing puts major emphasis on establishing relationships with physicians and encouraging them to make fuller use of hospital services. Should the organization become too supportive of patients at the expense of physicians, it risks alienating its source of economic livelihood. At the least, it will have apathetic or angry physicians. An obvious answer to this apparent dilemma is to make physicians part of the corporate culture. Then, the organizational philosophy and its principles become part of their perspective as well. They, too, will see substandard clinical treatment as endangering this culture, and work with the organization to be rid of the threat.

The view expressed by Williams and Donnelly is consistent with the high degree of trust the public places in health services organizations and an appropriate measure of the duty they should execute in turn. The public has every right to expect that the organization and those who manage it will treat them with respect and dignity. For many, this means being treated very differently from how they are treated now.

Relationship to Staff

Like patients, employees and medical staff are entitled to be treated with respect. They are the means by which the organization delivers services to patients. Like patients, employees should not be treated as a means to an end. The ethical aspects of these relations are most apparent in personnel policies officially or unofficially adopted by the organization. Examples include: reasonable and equitable evaluation standards that are known to personnel in advance and fairly applied; forthright efforts to eliminate capriciousness, arbitrariness, and prejudice in hiring, firing, and promotion; application of due process and access to a grievance procedure; and determining attributes and capabilities required for each position and matching personnel with them.[10] These considerations of ethics in employee relations also make good management sense.

Employees are not in an equal bargaining situation with supervisors— their freedom of action is limited by the employment relationship. For this reason, a manager who borrows money from employees behaves unethically. Not only does such an act jeopardize management credibility with employees, but more importantly, it reflects a lack of respect toward employees.

Medical staff are indispensable to most health services organizations. Whether they are independent contractors or salaried employees, their presence in the organization complicates its relationship with patients and nonmedical staff, since physicians may engage in activities that are at variance with the organizational philosophy. Medical staff who function as independent contractors cause unique management problems. If the organization is to perform its duties to the patient, it may have to intervene in the caregiver relationship. The organization's relationship to employees and medical staff can never be more important than its relationship with patients.

Employees and medical staff should participate in developing the organization's philosophy and mission statement. Increased congruence between the philosophies of organization and staff benefits the parties involved and, most importantly, benefits the patient. Rapport between the organization and its employees and medical staff is essential to developing the corporate culture described above.

Relationship to Community

In some geographic areas, community (service area) and patients are synonymous. In many other areas, this is not the case. The organization's philosophy should specify its relationship to the community. What is the organization's obligation to provide free or less than cost care to Medicaid patients or to the medically indigent? What is its obligation to provide controversial services, such as abortion? Posing and answering questions such as these causes the organization to address important questions about itself and its role prospectively. This is a useful exercise in honing an organizational philosophy, and also provides an opportunity for introspection and staff involvement in creating a corporate culture.

Relationship to Other Institutions

Developing and revising the organizational philosophy is increasingly difficult as competitive pressures mount. The organization must deal in a forthright and honest manner with all organizations, even those that may be current or future competitors. This ethic is compatible with effective competition. It simply means that the organization competes without fraud or deception. The organization relies on honest dealings to compete successfully. Although modest levels of cooperation have existed among health services organizations in the past, the future is likely to include less cooperation among organizations within the same service area, except insofar as they join multi-institutional systems.

Major differences in moral philosophies inhibit cooperative efforts. When Catholic health services organizations contemplate merger or joint efforts with non-Catholic organizations, abortion is a major stumbling block. When such mergers succeed, abortions and sterilization procedures are eliminated, or are performed only at facilities not legally linked to the new organization.

DEVELOPING A MISSION STATEMENT

Mission statements may originate in the organization's articles of incorporation, the documents filed to establish it as a legal entity. Sometimes they are stated as organizational objectives. The statement in the articles of incorporation of the purposes for which the corporation is established is also useful in developing a mission statement. In turn, the mission statement must be consistent with and reflect the organization's philosophy. A simple mission statement, stripped of excess verbiage, states that an acute care community hospital association will:

- Establish, operate, and maintain a hospital
- Engage in educational activities related to treating the sick and injured
- Engage in health promotion and disease prevention activities
- Promote and perform scientific research related to treating the sick and injured
- Engage in other activities designed to promote the general health of the community

More elaborate are the objectives (mission statement) of Sterling County Hospital. Here, elements of an organizational philosophy are included:

- To recognize man's unique composition of body and soul and man's basic right to life. Sterling County's concept of total care, therefore, embraces the physical, emotional, spiritual, social, and economic needs of each patient;
- To affirm that the primary objective of our health services is to relieve suffering and to promote and restore health in a Christian manner that demands competence, mercy, and respect;
- To generate and cultivate a source of allied health manpower by orienting and supporting personnel development in the areas of individual skills, knowledge, and attidues;
- To participate in the development of health services that are relevant to the total community needs by meaningful area-wide and regional planning and in a partnership for health concept.[11]

These mission statements show what the two organizations seek to do. An important distinction is that the first has no value context, nor is there any attempt to link its activities to a larger value system. The second is set within a philosophical context.

Organizations state their missions in a variety of ways. A well-known children's hospital states that it will provide health services to any child, regardless of ability to pay. This mission statement incorporates the philosophy that treating the child is the primary concern; economics are secondary. Organizations that are affiliated with a particular religion cite their religious creeds; non-sectarian organizations typically link their activities to humanitarian motives. (Sterling County Hospital is unique in that it is a public facility with a religious reference in its mission statement.)

RECONSIDERING THE ORGANIZATION'S PHILOSOPHY

The new competitive environment will have a significant effect on the way many health services organizations born of eleemosynary motives view themselves. Similarly, it will change how others, including patients and communities, see them. Competing aggressively for patients will be at variance with their historical philosophy and mission to serve the sick and injured, and to do so from a sense of duty and charity, rather than a desire to establish new product lines, increase market share, and improve net income over expense. The organization may not have the stamina, resources, or mindset to reconsider its philosophy and mission effectively. If so, it may become uneconomic and cease to exist. A case is illustrative.

An Acceptable New Image?

Sebastian Hospital was founded by a Christian congregation in 1891. Its philosophy and mission statements included a strong commitment to care for the sick and injured regardless of ability to pay. This mission posed no problems during the first 80 years of existence. Even after the hospital was purchased by the community in 1950, it continued to function in the same fashion. Sebastian Hospital successfully weathered a controversy about performing abortions in 1973. The compromise involved limiting where in the hospital abortions would be performed and how staff would be assigned to abortions.

Increasing cost pressures on the hospital during the 1970s, and DRG reimbursement in the early 1980s, began to cause substantial financial problems. All-payor prospective payment, which would prohibit cost shifting, was imminent. In addition, there were presssures for corporate reorganization. A report from planning consultants recommended undertaking enterprises such as physician office buildings, parking facilities, and a motel. Some of these were complementary to the primary mission of caring for the sick and injured. Others were seen by the trustees as tangential. Now, yet another new type of enterprise is being proposed—a joint venture with members of the medical staff.

The administrator was concerned that the focus of the hospital for almost 100 years would change dramatically. It was one thing to manage a facility competently, but quite another to be razzle-dazzle entrepreneurs. Would the caring aspect that Sebastian had achieved so well disappear in a blaze of marketing and joint ventures? The administrator wondered whether the organization wasn't hopelessly out of step with its environment.

This case illustrates the dilemma confronting a typical not-for-profit community hospital. The same or similar problems affect most organizations in the sense that they must continue to adapt to the sometimes dramatic changes occurring in the environment. Interinstitutional competition is less problematic when there is one of each type of institutional provider in a community. Even here, however, to broaden their range of activities, institutions may begin to offer services that impinge on other institutions' traditional territory. Furthermore, physicians are likely to undertake development of free-standing outpatient services, such as surgicenters and diagnostic facilities. If, for example, physicians perform highly remunerative ancillary and diagnostic services outside hospitals—something increasingly permitted by technology—existing organizations may lose substantial revenue. This will exacerbate the pressure to compete aggressively in a market that now includes its own medical staff as competitors. Such tensions may diminish the hospital's ability to carry out its mission within its historical philosophy.

For many in the not-for-profit sector, widespread use of the term *marketing* in the health services field conjures up images of persons of questionable ethics selling unneeded items of little value. They prefer health services organizations to limit their activities to health promotion and disease and accident prevention and treatment. Yet, marketing is the new watchword, and failure to heed it puts organizations at financial risks.

The need to compete is not at variance with the mission to provide charity services. The context has changed and the stakes are higher, but these changes should be viewed by managers as a challenge—an opportunity to do what they have been doing, but more effectively. Successful corporate restructuring and marketing activities permit the organization to develop the sources of income that enable it to provide charity services.

A more insidious problem—and one with major potential for conflicts of interest—is presented by some manifestations of joint ventures between health services organizations, especially hospitals, and medical staffs. Physicians whose income is in whole or in part dependent on referring patients to facilities in which they have personally invested or where they have a profit-sharing arrangement have a conflict of interests. The physician's economic tie to the organization is often concealed, and states such as Michigan, Pennsylvania, and California have either prohibited physician referral to such facilities or have mandated disclosure of that information to patients. Organized medicine has begun to take note of these types of conflicts of interests.[12]

Another kind of philosophical dilemma faced St. Joseph Hospital. Established in 1870, St. Joseph's was owned by various orders of Catholic sisters until 1971, when it was sold to the Creighton Regional Health Care Corporation, a not-for-profit corporation with a lay board of directors. This board continued to operate St. Joseph as a Catholic teaching hospital for Creighton University. In 1984, a contract was signed with American Medical International (AMI), a for-profit hospital system, under which AMI would acquire St. Joseph Hospital and operate it as a full-service Catholic teaching hospital. Based on this transfer of ownership, the Catholic Health Association (CHA) terminated St. Joseph's membership because "the Hospital is not operated, supervised, or controlled by or in conjunction with the Roman Catholic Church in the United States."[13] The controversy surrounding the decision suggested that other important, but unstated, reasons were questions about the morality of the profit motive in health services, and the fact that other hospitals in the AMI system performed abortions. Those challenging CHA's action argued that the profit motive was compatible with St. Joseph's mission, and that bondholders of St. Joseph's debt were paid several millions of dollars in interest—an action said to be indistinguishable from that of paying dividends to stockholders.

What is important here is the fact that CHA determined that certain actions taken by a member hospital were incompatible with its philosophy and mission, and took action. Whether or not CHA's action was morally right or wrong, the point to be made is that its decision was based on a specific philosophy—a crucial underpinning for any organization.

PATIENT BILLS OF RIGHTS

A patient bill of rights provides guidance about the appropriate ethical relationship between the patient on the one hand and the organization and its employees on the other. Titles vary, but bills of rights have been published by organizations including the American Hospital Association (AHA), the Joint Commission on Accreditation of Healthcare Organizations (JCAHO), the Department of Veterans Affairs (DVA), and the American Civil Liberties Union (ACLU). In addition, hospitals and other institutional providers have developed individual statements. The AHA bill of patient rights is more oriented to institutional needs; its philosophy is quite different from that of the ACLU. The DVA's Code of Patient Concern and the JCAHO's Rights and Responsibilities of Patients lie somewhere between the two. As the name suggests, the JCAHO statement includes a section on the responsibilities of patients in cooperating with caregivers.

All patient bills of rights reflect the law on matters such as confidentiality and consent. The ACLU bill of rights is much more demanding—almost strident—in its view of patients' rights than are the other bills, especially the AHA bill. The ACLU bill mandates an advocate for each patient and total access by patients to their medical records while hospitalized, and provision of a copy of those records upon discharge. It also specifies in detail the content of information to be provided when obtaining consent for treatment. The ACLU statement views the patient as an autonomous individual entitled to full involvement in the care process. It even suggests that the patient has a duty to be fully involved. Its stridency is unconventional, yet it contains points worth considering in developing an organization's philosophy.

Provisions in the AHA version suggest a distinct element of paternalism. The AHA recognizes that there may be times when patients should not be fully informed of their medical condition. This reflects a paternalistic philosophy rooted in medical ethical tradition dating to the Hippocratic Oath, and puts the desire to do good (beneficence) in conflict with enhancing the patient's autonomy.

Although some provisions of these bills of patient rights reflect the law, no patient bill of rights is itself legally binding. Such documents set an ethical tone as to how the patient is to be treated, and serve as a nonformal source of law if a dispute arises. The usefulness of such documents is limited by the organization's willingness to adopt one already available or develop its own, and, more importantly, to implement the bill of rights by making its contents known to patients and monitoring processes that show their application.

STRATEGIC PLANNING

The organization's philosophy also affects its strategic planning. The philosophy must be articulated if planning objectives are to be consistent, as well as appropriately set. The organization's view of its social responsibility should be reflected in both the organizational philosophy and mission statement. Once philosophy and mission are established, the strategic planning process can proceed.

It is widely accepted that an organization's philosophy and mission are statements of ideals—ends thought to be unattainable but progress toward which is believed possible.[14] In this respect, perhaps the most difficult aspect of developing a strategy is determining the balance between social responsibility and economic performance.[15] Resolving this dilemma and the paradoxes it raises will be more difficult in the future. While an organization's governing body is primarily responsible for developing its philosophy and the resulting mission statement, the planning process and development of specific operational plans based on it are the responsibility of senior management. Consistency between the organization's philosophy and its specific procedures and rules must be maintained.

CONGRUENCE OF PHILOSOPHIES

Several questions must be asked about the relationship between the manager's personal ethic and the organization's philosophy. To what extent is it necessary that organizational philosophy and the personal ethic of managers mesh? For the organization to become a community of shared values, is it necessary that all members of management be in total agreement with the philosophy? As a class, are managers sufficiently professional that they can effectively manage an organization with whose values they may partly disagree? What degree of congruence is needed? A literal reading of Deal and Kennedy suggests that philosophical divergence should be discouraged and all values must be shared by all employees, including managers.

Some health services organizations require that all managers at midlevel and above be members of the same religious faith as that of the sponsoring group. Apparently, they judge their philosophy and mission to be unique, so that only coreligionists can effectively manage their organizations. Some philosophies are unique, but such a requirement seems excessive in most settings and situations. If this policy breeds conformity and diminishes innovation, it is also counterproductive.

As part of their interview and pre-employment processes, organizations should determine the potential manager's personal ethic about health services delivery, and explain their own philosophy. This permits both parties to judge the extent of their philosophical congruence. This should be done whether or not the individual under consideration is a coreligionist, because even among persons of the same faith there may be significantly divergent views. Similarly, organizations with a humanist or humanitarian philosophy, whether publicly or privately owned, may not want to employ persons whose ethic constrains them from participating in certain services (e.g., abortion). Here, too, such information can and should be known prospectively.

In such situations, it should be remembered that persons may reach the same conclusions about a sectarian organization's appropriate role and its relationship to patients by relying on a moral philosophy and principles that are not linked to the organization's religious doctrine. Such managers would be effective in working to achieve the same goals as others in the organization because, as Deal and Kennedy stress, they share the same values. The measure should be congruence between the organization's philosophy and the results of a manager's decision making as well as other indications. Someone claiming moral neutrality is potentially the most inimical to an organization seeking to implement an organizational philosophy and develop a corporate culture.

CONCLUSION

This chapter describes the importance of the organizational philosophy in determining an organization's mission. From philosophy and mission are derived policies and procedures—the stuff from which the abstract and sometimes elusive aspects of the organization are operationalized. Developing a corporate culture is a desirable result of shared values. And while shared values are important in easing discontinuity and achieving corporate effectiveness, there is a school of behavioral thought that suggests that the unwillingness of those who disagree to speak out is a major source of problems in organizations. This type of problem is exacerbated if the organization becomes an environment of group think.

A variety of sources assists in developing an organization's philosophy. These include religious affiliation or orientation and humanism or humanitarian motives. Employee and patient bills of rights are others. Whatever sources an organization draws on, the principles of respect for persons, beneficence, non-maleficence, and justice must be included.

NOTES

1. Thomas J. Peters and Robert H. Waterman, Jr., *In Search of Excellence: Lessons from America's Best-Run Companies* (New York: Harper & Row, 1982), 15.

2. Terrence E. Deal and Allan A. Kennedy, *Corporate Cultures: The Rites and Rituals of Corporate Life* (Reading, MA: Addison-Wesley Publishing Co., 1982).

3. Deal and Kennedy, *Corporate Cultures,* 22.

4. Allan A. Kennedy, "Corporate Values/Corporate Culture." In *Excellence in Management: Lessons Learned from Other Industries,* report from a special conference for American College of Hospital Administrators Fellows, October 29–30, 1985, 5–7.

5. Terrence E. Deal, Allan A. Kennedy, and Arthur H. Spiegel, III, "How to Create An Outstanding Hospital Culture," *Hospital Forum 27* (January/February 1983): 21–28, 33–34.

6. Peters and Waterman, *Excellence,* 15–16.

7. Philosophy of the Franciscan Health System, 1986; Mission Statement, Saint Mary Hospital, Langhorne, Pennsylvania.

8. Ibid.

9. Kenneth J. Williams and Paul R. Donnelly, *Medical Care Quality and the Public Trust* (Chicago: Pluribus Press, 1982).

10. Bonnie J. Gray and Robert K. Landrum, "Difficulties With Being Ethical," *Business 33* (July–September 1983): 28–33.

11. Ed D. Roach and Bobby G. Bizzell, "Sterling County Hospital." In *Cases in Health Services Management,* edited by Jonathon S. Rakich, Beaufort B. Longest, Jr., and Kurt Darr (Baltimore: Health Professions Press, 1990), 144.

12. "Dealing with Conflicts of Interest," Editorial, *New England Journal of Medicine 313* (September 1985): 749–751.

13. Richard L. O'Brien and Michael J. Haller, "Investor-Owned or Nonprofit?" *New England Journal of Medicine 313* (July 1985): 198–201.

14. R.L. Ackoff, *Creating the Corporate Future* (New York: John Wiley & Sons, 1981).

15. James Webber, "Planning," *Hospitals 56* (April 1, 1982): 69–70.

4

∞

CODES OF ETHICS IN HEALTH SERVICES

M ANY FACTORS INFLUENCE HUMAN BEHAVIOR and interaction. Among the most basic are those that arise from the individual's legal relationships with society—the increasingly pervasive laws, ordinances, regulations, and court rulings. Other types of formal rules, such as the bylaws governing a private organization, apply only to the organization itself. The link between formal sources of law and ethics was described in the Introduction. In addition, there are nonformal sources of laws, such as standards of justice, public policies, moral convictions, customary laws, and notions of individual equity. Both formal and nonformal sources of law are used by private associations such as health services organizations. Codes of ethics adopted by a professional organization are significant because they state the organization's goals, guide its affiliates, and in turn serve as a reference point to discipline those who deviate from the norms.

In 1978, federal law created the Office of Government Ethics to review activities of certain executive branch officials to determine whether they were in conflict with their public duties. The law was reauthorized for 6 years in 1988. As amended, it provides for, among other things, financial disclosure by designated persons; restriction of certain activities after such persons leave government service; restrictions on gifts from outside sources; and restrictions on outside earned income, honoraria, and outside employment (financial interests that are deemed too remote or inconsequential to affect the integrity of services are exempt). The office's main source of information is the annual individual financial disclosure statement. States have comparable statutes. For affected employees, these laws are important sources of ethical and legal guidance.

A 1984 survey by the public interest group Common Cause of 50 officials designated by federal agencies as "ethics officers" found that only a few spent more than 15% of their time on ethics-related matters. The report was generally critical of the way in which ethics are enforced, and noted that the most frequently ignored regulations had to do with limitations on contact between employees and the agencies at which they formerly worked.[1]

Historically, self-regulation has been one of the hallmarks of the learned professions (law, medicine, and the clergy). Their ethics are reflected in bar discipline, principles of medical ethics, and ecclesiastic law. As law, medicine, and other, newer professions sought regulation (protection) through legislation or had such legislation forced on them, many of their ethical principles were incorporated into statutes or regulations, or, in the case of lawyers, court-adopted disciplinary guidelines.

Any group seeking professional status should have a code of ethics. Codes are common in health services, and most managerial and technical groups have them. Their language is usually general, and performance standards are usually vague to the point that fair enforcement is impossible. In the latter regard, attorneys represent a notable exception. A wag might suggest that this is as it should be, since lawyers seem to have a disproportionate share of ethics problems. Lawyers are officers of the court, and have a positive duty to report information that raises substantial questions about another lawyer's honesty, trustworthiness, or fitness. Their principles of ethics have judicial sanction, because typically the highest court in the state adopts (with few modifications) the Code of Professional Responsibility of the American Bar Association (a private association) as the state rules of professional conduct. The court usually appoints a board of professional responsibility to enforce the rules and to review and investigate complaints, which are heard by a special panel of judges. Adverse action by this panel results in penalties ranging from admonition or probation to suspension or revocation of the attorney's license. The bar association is very important because of its role in developing the code of conduct that reflects the profession's ethics.

It is clear, however, that even with reasonably stringent enforcement, the major purpose of a code of ethics is to guide the behavior and decisions of persons who want to do the right thing but need help determining what that is. The individual who is trying to get away with something will always be at the fringe of a profession. Principles of ethical conduct (and legal requirements, as well) will serve only to encourage such people to avoid being caught. Even absent codes of ethics, however, certain actions will raise questions about the character of an individual.

Mr. B

Mr. B sought a new position as a consultant in health services. He contacted two firms and was interviewed by both. One offered him a position. Mr. B verbally accepted the job, even though it meant moving. Several days later, as a courtesy, he called the second firm to tell them he had taken a position. The managing partner said, "Gee, that's really too bad, I was going to offer you a job in your area and pay you $5,000 more than you got from the other firm."

Mr. B has an ethical problem. He verbally accepted the position, and even though there is no written contract, he gave his word that he would take the first offer. If Mr. B were to call the first firm and explain what happened, they would probably release him—they would not want to hire a disgruntled employee. This does not affect his ethical obligation to take the job offer he accepted, however. Having made the commitment, Mr. B is morally bound to meet it.

CODES FOR MANAGERS

In addition to what those in the profession consider minimally appropriate behavior, codes also state the profession's goals and objectives. These goals may be unachievable, but the profession must nonetheless work toward them, since considerable progress is often achievable. These are important dimensions of codes of ethics, which, like the philosophy and mission statements, are developed by health services organizations.

Research involving business students suggests that ethics can be taught and learned, but that after a period of time (4 years, in one study) lack of reinforcement causes graduates to be no better prepared than they were before they took an ethics course.[2] The implication is that continuing education in ethics for health services managers is essential.

Code for Health Services Managers

The most prominent health services management group is the American College of Healthcare Executives (ACHE), known before mid-1985 as the American College of Hospital Administrators (ACHA). In 1990, it had over 23,000 affiliates.

The ACHE (ACHA) has had a code of ethics since 1939, 6 years after its founding. Initially, it was linked to the code of ethics for hospitals developed by the American Hospital Association (AHA). In the ensuing iterations, however, the ACHE's code has become increasingly distinct; it has also become more explicit. The current code was adopted in 1988. The emphasis is on ethical issues in management, including conflict of interest, confidential information, and governing body and medical staff relations. The 1988 Code of Ethics is reproduced in Appendix B.

Historically, the code has paid no attention to biomedical ethical issues. This orientation is reflected in the 1988 version, although the new code includes a statement on life continuation decisions. Little attention is paid to patients' rights and the independent duty owed by managers to patients. The ACHE code has not attempted to define the limits of loyalty (fidelity) to the organization and the point at which that loyalty is superseded by a duty to the patient. This is a vital facet of the manager's role as a moral agent.

Important changes in the 1988 code are: specific reference to resource allocation, specific reference to the manager's responsibility for ethical behavior in advertising, and inclusion of a provision that affiliates are obligated to bring to the ethics committee information about code violations. This latter change is critical for building esprit de corps among ACHE affiliates and making the code a living document with clear application in management practice.

Actions taken against affiliates under the code are highly structured and emphasize due process. The ACHE's committee on ethics receives complaints about allegedly unethical conduct. After informing the respondent (the affiliate), it refers the matter to the regent of the geographic area in which the respondent is presently employed. The regent investigates and reports to the committee. If the respondent appeals, or further investigation is necessary, the ACHE chairman appoints an ad hoc committee of three fellows from the region in which the respondent was employed when the alleged infraction occurred. This ad hoc committee hears the matter and sends a report, with recommendations, to the committee on ethics. Upon request, the respondent may make a personal appearance before the committee. This is considered an appeals hearing. After that hearing, the committee makes a decision and reports to the board of governors. The final review available to the respondent is before the board of governors.

The lengthy grievance and appeals procedure is designed to meet the criterion of fairness. It is also consistent with the trend toward applying legal requirements of procedural and substantive due process, even for private associations. The respondent can seek review of these decisions in the courts, but, historically, courts have been reluctant to review actions of private associations.

The maximum disciplinary action the board of governors can take against an affiliate is expulsion. ACHE affiliation is not linked to licensure and, therefore, disciplinary action by the ACHE has significance only if affiliation is important to colleagues and potential employers. If so, the former affiliate's employment and career opportunities become more limited. Future employers may be particularly interested in the reason for the disciplinary action. A policy question the ACHE should address is: What use is to be made of such information when affiliation in a professional association is voluntary?

In critiquing the 1973 version of the code, ACHE affiliates indicated that a code of ethics was important to them. They thought the code should be more comprehensive and more specific in guiding decision making on ethical problems. Moreover, more emphasis was believed to be needed on enforcement and on reporting to affiliates the disposition of cases, without naming the individuals involved. Affiliates also wanted to learn more about ethical problems.[3] A living code is more useful to affiliates as they confront ethical issues and work to solve them.

Code for Nursing Home Administrators

The Code of Ethics of the American College of Health Care Administrators (ACHCA) applies to its affiliates, who are primarily managers of long-term care facilities. The 1989 code is the latest version. It is reproduced in Appendix B.

Affiliates are expected to meet four "expectations," which are divided into prescriptions and proscriptions. These expectations state that: 1) the welfare of those for whom care is provided is paramount; 2) the affiliate shall maintain high levels of professional competence; 3) in all matters relating to their professional functions, the affiliate shall maintain a professional posture that makes paramount the interests of the facility and its residents; and 4) affiliates must honor their responsibilities to the public, profession, and other colleagues. Examples of issues receiving specific attention include: quality of services; confidentiality of patient information; continuing education; conflicts of interest; fostering knowledge, supporting research, and sharing expertise; and providing information to the standards and ethics committee of actual or potential code violations.

This latter requirement suggests a disciplinary process, but no enforcement or appeals processes are described. The preamble to the code states that the ultimate responsibility for applying standards and ethics falls on the individual. The ACHCA code pays even less attention to biomedical ethical issues than does the ACHE code—an important lapse for both groups.

CODES FOR CAREGIVERS

Codes for Physicians

The origins of ethics in medicine date from the Code of Hammurabi in the eighteenth century B.C. It established a payment schedule for treatments by physicians and veterinarians. The punishments indicated when a patient was harmed were harsh: a physician could lose his hands if the patient's eye or life was lost as a result of treatment.

A quite different code developed from the teaching and work of Hippocrates, who lived from about 460 to 370 B.C. Unlike the Code of Hammurabi, which was imposed by a ruler, the Hippocratic philosophy about relationships among physicians and between physicians and patients was developed by Greek physicians, one of whom could have been Hippocrates, for their own use. The Hippocratic Oath had no public sanction or force of law. It established standards of conduct, many of which have been incorporated into state licensing and regulation of physicians.

The Hippocratic Oath contains a lengthy section describing the appropriate relationship between physicians and their teachers and students—provisions that are largely obsolete. Other provisions no longer universally applied include restrictions on performing surgery, on assisting in abortion, and on applying dietetic measures to benefit the sick. Provisions prohibiting aiding in a suicide and refraining from sexual misconduct with patients and others in the household, and broad restrictions on confidentiality of any information learned during the course of medical treatment continue to be reflected in the current medical code, specifically or by implication. They are also used in state licensing.

The American Medical Association (AMA) was founded in 1847. Its first code of medical ethics was based on the work of Thomas Percival, the English physician, philosopher, and writer. Its ethics code has been revised several times; the most recent edition of the Principles of Medical Ethics, reproduced in Appendix B, was adopted in 1980. The previous version, adopted in 1957, was more proscriptive. It prohibited advertising and proscribed voluntary association with practitioners who have no scientific basis for treatment. The most significant change, however, is philosophical, and affects the relationship between physician and patient. Previous versions of the code included a distinct element of paternalism—physicians could act in ways that they considered to be in the patient's best interests. Although the 1980 principles do not reflect a covenant or contract between patient and physician, the profession seems to be moving in that direction. Veatch states: "It is the first document in the history of professional medical ethics in which a group of physicians is willing to use the language of responsibilities and rights," rather than that of benefits and harms.[4]

AMA members have a positive duty to ". . . strive to expose those physicians deficient in character or competence, or who engage in fraud or deception."[5] This statement's directiveness and specificity are unique among codes for caregivers, and it sets a philosophical tone for the profession. Critics argue that this duty has been widely ignored.

To assist members in understanding how the principles are applied, the AMA's Judicial Council publishes opinions that interpret the code with regard to issues such as experimentation, genetic engineering, abortion, and terminal illness. These opinions are very useful in supplementing the Principles.

Code for Nurses

The Code for Nurses promulgated by the American Nurses Association (ANA) was first adopted in 1950. The 1985 version, reproduced in Appendix B, is the most recent. The preamble states that clients are the primary decision makers in matters concerning their own health, treatment, and well-being, and "the goal of nursing actions is to support the client's responsibility and self-determination to the greatest extent possible."[6] This is a philosophy without a hint of paternalism.

Also included in the preamble is a list of the principles that are expected to govern interactions with clients. These principles are similar to those identified in Chapter 2. The introduction states that the code "serves to inform both the nurse and society of the profession's expectations and requirements in ethical matters."[7]

The code has 11 provisions, many of which are quite specific. Each is followed by an interpretative statement. One provision is similar to the AMA requirement that the caregiver has a positive duty to expose unethical or incompetent practice. It states that "the nurse acts to safeguard the client and the public when health care and safety are affected by the incompetent, unethical, or illegal practice of any person."[8]

CODES FOR INSTITUTIONS

Code for Hospitals

The American Hospital Association (AHA) is the most important trade association for hospitals. It adopted revised guidelines for ethical conduct in 1987. These guidelines are divided into community role, patient care, and organizational conduct. Members are expected to improve community health status and deliver high-quality, comprehensive services efficiently. Emphasis is put on the importance of coordination with other health services organizations. Some provisions are specific: the need for informed consent; for confidentiality; and for mechanisms to resolve conflicting values among patients and families, medical staff, employees, the organization, and the community. Members must try to accommodate the religious and social beliefs and customs of patients, but they do not override the organization's own creed. The guidelines identify expectations regarding employees in terms of employee policies and practices and accommodation of the religious and moral values held by employees and medical staff, and define conflicts of interest.

Codes for Nursing Facilities (NFs)

The American Health Care Association (AHCA) is the national association that serves long-term care facilities, primarily nursing facilities (NFs). It does not have a specific code of ethics. Members are expected to abide by the patient bill of rights adopted by the institution. The patient bill of rights specifies that there should be a balancing of rights, and enumerates those rights for patients in long-term care facilities. These rights are especially concerned with fair treatment, information, communication, choice, and privacy—on minimizing the dehumanizing aspects of institutional care. Some state laws require NFs receiving Medicaid funds to follow a patients' bill of rights based on that of the AHCA.

The American Association of Homes for the Aging (AAHA) is the national association that represents not-for-profit homes, housing, health-related facilities, and community services for the elderly. It has no specific code of ethics, but in 1988 its task force on ethics issued a white paper whose purpose is to enhance the capability of members to "do ethics" at the corporate level. Substantive issues addressed include treatment decisions, decision-making capacity of patients and surrogate decision making, the autonomy of residents, admission and discharge policy, internal corporate issues, external corporate issues, research, and social activism. Procedural issues addressed include decision making, organization, and financial administration (planning, budgeting, etc.).

PHILOSOPHICAL BASES FOR CODES OF ETHICS

Modern ethics codes for the health professions blend deontological and consequentialist philosophies in their assumptions and underpinnings. To varying extents, the principles of respect for persons, beneficence, nonmaleficence, and justice are found in all of the codes described.

In both the ACHE and ACHCA codes, there is a blending of deontological and consequentialist elements, although the emphasis is on the deontological. The principles of respect for persons and beneficence are prominent. The ACHE section on conflict of interest, for example, assumes that there is an independent right action. Except for the reference that "a conflict of interest may be only a matter of degree," the action itself, rather than the results (consequences) of the action, is reviewed in determining moral rightness or wrongness. Similarly, the statements on confidential information are deontological—no weighing of consequences is permitted.

New in the 1988 ACHE code is the duty to report violations: "An affiliate of the College who has reasonable grounds to believe another affiliate has violated this Code has a duty to communicate such facts to the Committee on Ethics."[9] The 1989 ACHCA code has a similar provision.

The 1980 AMA Principles included a new view of physician duty and respect for patients. The preamble provides the context: "A physician must recognize responsibility not only to patients, but also to society, to other health professionals, and to self."[10] This philosophy is absent in the Hippocratic Oath and the 1957 version of the AMA Principles. There the emphasis was paternalistic—there was no suggestion that the patient's interests had to be balanced against the interests of society. This change has implications for resource allocation decisions. Furthermore, it suggests that the effect on society of the costs of individual treatment decisions should be considered. This philosophy is based on the principle of justice, rather than the principle of beneficence, which focuses on patients. This adds a dimension of utilitarianism, which considers the greatest good for the greatest number.

The ANA Code for Nurses is more heavily deontological than the other codes examined here. Within this philosophical context, respect for persons and beneficence clearly undergird the relationship with clients.

APPLYING CODES OF ETHICS

Enforcement

Codes of ethics take on real meaning when they are enforced. Unenforced they represent mere platitudes intended for public consumption, and are only marginally useful to the profession. Enforceable codes must be sufficiently precise, or include comprehensive interpretations of their provisions. Absent sufficient detail to guide the affiliate, enforcement results in arbitrary decision making and denial of due process. As noted earlier, private associations are not usually held to constitutional requirements of due process, but it is fair (just) that they should meet such a standard nonetheless. This theme should underlie an organization's relationships with affiliates. Enforcement with feedback to affiliates provides additional knowledge and understanding for the profession, and makes the code a living document. This attribute is critical.

Enforcement of codes is typically achieved through a grievance procedure. The procedure prescribed for the ACHE puts great emphasis on procedural due process—it seeks to be eminently fair to the grievant. Appeals are heard privately, and no information is communicated to affiliates that are not directly involved. Even when the affiliate's unethical activity is also the subject of a criminal proceeding and conviction, the ACHE does not identify the respondent.

The public scrutiny that results from licensing health services professionals usually means that actions on licensure status are a matter of public record. Reports of disciplinary actions against physicians appear regularly in the press. Actions against attorneys are also a matter of public record.

Except for nursing home administrators, health services managers have no licensing requirements. However, scandals could lead to demands for licensure—a less desirable means of regulating conduct than voluntary self-regulation. This suggests the special importance of voluntary efforts, and the need to enforce usable, living (interpreted) codes of ethics.

A major aspect of a code of ethics is its process of providing information feedback to affiliates, especially information about interpretation, application, and enforcement. There is also need for general education to apprise affiliates of code provisions and changes. Few efforts have been directed at making health services administrative or institutional codes living documents actively used in guiding decision making, however. Health services administrators, especially those with little experience, are interested in learning about the code of ethics that guides their professional association.[11] Finding means to encourage and respond to this interest remains an important, but unmet, challenge to the profession.

Separating Private and Public Actions

Managers of health services organizations are public figures. The community's interest in them and their organizations is reflected in their importance in the community. A manager's role outside the organization is greater in small communities, where the organization, especially the acute care hospital, is economically, politically, and socially important. This means that health services managers are often community leaders, and thus live in a fishbowl. In urban areas as well, managers of major health services organizations are considered community leaders because of their positions. Managers must be prepared to accept this public trust and confidence, and use it to improve the community's health. However, playing such a role requires a high standard of performance.

It is difficult to determine the point at which a prominent person can escape public scrutiny and claim privacy. It may be that prominent persons never escape public scrutiny. This is especially difficult for younger, less experienced managers to understand. They jealously guard their privacy. Most consider their conduct in their personal lives irrelevant to their performance as managers. Yet their role in the organization and the public's expectations of them do not permit them this luxury.

The dynamic between the manager's public and private life is affected by three elements: 1) the corrupt moral standard that the absolute right or wrong of an act is less important than whether one is caught, 2) the organization's culture and the community standard of behavior and morality, and 3) administrative effectiveness. "It's okay if you don't get caught" or "It's okay, everybody's doing it" are unacceptable standards for health services managers. To appreciate the effect of such views, even simple applications are instructive. Most persons would be embarrassed to be seen photocopying personal papers at their place of employment, or to have personal long-distance phone calls that were made at the organization's expense brought to the attention of their superiors. Wasted time, personal use of office equipment, and personal phone calls will not result in disciplinary action by a professional association, nor, in all likelihood, by the organization. Such actions must be regulated by the individual's personal ethic. Members of the profession should consider even these small infractions to be governed by the principles developed in Chapter 1, as well as the standards in professional codes of conduct.

The organization's culture and the community standard of morality are important because to a large extent the community and the organization's culture affect managers' views of acceptable and unacceptable behavior. This is tempered by the individual's personal ethic.

In addition to the community at large, there is the microcommunity, the corporate culture, discussed in Chapter 3. The mores and standards developed by these microcosms are unique and demanding. They are ignored at one's peril.

It Just Isn't Done!

Several university faculty members had the opportunity to have lunch with a group of 20 middle and senior managers of a data-processing firm. It was an enthusiastic and highly motivated group, most of whom were less than 40 years of age. Lunch was a break in a long day of seminars and meetings. When the waiter asked around the table for drink orders, no member of the firm ordered an alcoholic beverage. Instead, they ordered milk or soda. One of the faculty members who remarked about this unusual behavior was told it was an unwritten company policy that no member of the staff should have a drink and go back to work.

This may seem a bit straitlaced. It is certainly different from the two martinis once considered the norm for business lunches. Yet this rule reflected the group's self-view (culture), and substantial peer pressure would likely be directed at those behaving differently. Whether on a macro or a micro scale, this is the type of peer pressure that a group such as health services managers can exercise for the good of the patient and the profession.

Administrative effectiveness is most important for the manager's supervisor, who must ask, have the problems fatally flawed the manager's ability to lead? At some point, a manager's reputation may become badly tarnished; eventually, such managers lose their effectiveness. If the manager is ridiculed, if the character deficit is blatant and known to all, if respect is eroded or gone, then the manager's supervisor must fire the manager.

It may seem unfair that managers are held to a higher standard than the community at large. Employees and the public expect more of leaders than they do of followers. The health services profession correctly expects its members to avoid the temptations and problems affecting those outside it.

Another example of private behavior that is considered unacceptable in a health services manager is drunk driving. Regardless of the view taken by professional groups, governing bodies have little tolerance for managers who drive while intoxicated, although such behavior on the part of a housekeeping worker would likely go unpunished. Driving while intoxicated runs counter to the organization's philosophy, which for problems such as alcohol and drug abuse, illicit sexual activity, and spouse abuse, will be unwritten. Activities that are illegal are considered unethical per se. They are not explicitly prohibited only because the governing body considers them so obviously unacceptable.

Another reason such behavior is considered unacceptable is that the governing body does not want to be embarrassed by an errant manager. An organization faced with scandal will act to separate itself from the source of unacceptable behavior. This reaction reflects the instinctive urge for organizational survival, as well as indignation and moral revulsion. Major problems occur, however, in attempting to instill in others an awareness of the importance of ethical behavior in an organization.

Is This a Laughing Matter?

One afternoon, Joan Zimmerman, the chief operating officer of a large hospital, encountered two younger members of her management staff conversing in hushed tones. As Zimmerman approached unnoticed, they burst into laughter. One of the two blushed and turned his eyes downward as Zimmerman greeted them and asked lightheartedly about the source of their amusement. At first, neither spoke. Sensing there was something she should know, Zimmerman pressed for an answer.

The awkward situation was interrupted by Zimmerman's pager, which asked her to call the operator immediately. Later, one of the two asked to see Zimmerman. He related an amazing story about the female director of one of the support departments. Apparently, the personnel department had been investigating the reasons for the high turnover rate in that department. In exit interviews, several young male employees claimed that they were leaving because they could no longer endure the sexual harassment by the department's director, who insisted that the young men have sex with her. Those who did not were penalized professionally. Zimmerman was told that the problem had existed for some time, and was an open secret throughout the hospital. Zimmerman was shocked and very distressed that she had not known about it.

This case has several dimensions. First and most importantly, sexual harrassment is against the law. Second, sexual harrassment breaches the principle of respect for persons. Third, the unfair treatment of staff by the department head breaches the principle of justice.

Also of concern is that the younger managers found the case amusing, rather than outrageous. Their reaction may indicate a lack of maturity rather than the view that the behavior is not unethical. This problem needs attention, as does the more immediate one of what to do about the department head. Managers lead by actions and words, and actions are the more important.

Two other problems are that Zimmerman herself was not aware of the problem, and that there was a lack of action by those who were aware. If correct, the allegations cast a shadow on all managers and the organization itself. Zimmerman must make it clear to all employees that such behavior is intolerable. It breaches the trust placed in management staff and is inconsistent with any organizational philosophy worthy of the name.

CONCLUSION

Most codes of ethics provide only general guidelines. Even specific provisions must be interpreted and applied. Interpretation is crucial, since even great detail cannot address the nuances and intricacies of various situations. A detailed code would be excessively legalistic, and applying it would be a nightmare.

Of the professional groups in health services management, the ACHE has developed the most detailed code. This makes it useful as a guide to health services managers, whether or not they are ACHE affiliates. The code is, nonetheless, too general to provide performance standards.

The AMA's Principles are useful because the Judicial Council interprets the principles and their application. Comparison of the ACHE and AMA codes suggests that the ACHE Code of Ethics has become more explicit and the AMA Principles of Medical Ethics less so as they evolved.

Codes in the health services field carry only the sanctions that can be applied by the professional association. The maximum discipline is expulsion. This is unlikely to affect the individual's legal right to engage in the profession.

In addition to the ethical codes of their private professional associations, virtually all clinical groups are regulated by state law. Licensure statutes—or practice acts as they are often called—incorporate many of the same ethical principles as the professional group. This is to be expected, since licensing boards are usually composed of members of the profession being regulated. This gives ethical precepts of the profession the force of law—breaching them could lead to license suspension or revocation. It is noteworthy that the proceedings of public regulators are distinct from those of private associations or professional groups. Proper licensure is a condition of membership in the professional association, but membership in the association is not required for licensure.

For groups such as hospital managers, the lack of licensure places increased significance on how well it regulates itself. The public looks to the profession as the primary actor in safeguarding its health services system. Unless self-regulation is effective and sustains the public's confidence, licensing or another form of governmental regulation will result.

Another pragmatic consideration is the personal success of managers. A survey of leading hospital CEOs showed integrity to be the personality trait rated most important to success. Integrity was considered more important than any skill, or other trait or factor.[12] This additional stimulus to be ethical in all aspects of their lives should make health services managers more vigilant about themselves and their colleagues. These are significant reasons for maintaining the public's trust in health services managers and their organizations.

Far more critical than these pragmatic reasons for demanding ethical behavior is that ethical behavior is the right thing to do—it is a principle for life and the profession. The slightest hint of impropriety in personal behavior should be avoided. What a tragedy for the late Hyman G. Rickover, father of the nuclear fleet and a retired U.S. Navy admiral with an astounding 64 years on active duty, to have to admit that he took gifts from defense contractors. Rickover claimed that the gifts were trinkets, and that taking them did not affect his judgment. The Secretary of the Navy insisted that the gifts were worth tens of thousands of dollars. Whatever the facts, these revelations badly, and sadly, tarnished a distinguished career. It is just such situations that health services managers must assiduously avoid. Failing this, they risk their careers and reputations, and violate the principles of a personal ethic.

NOTES

1. Pete Earley, "Ethics Laws Found to be Laxly Enforced," *Washington Post,* November 30, 1984.

2. Peter Arlow and Thomas A. Ulrich, "Can Ethics Be Taught to Business Students?" *Collegiate Forum* (Spring 1983): 17.

3. Kurt Darr, "Administrative Ethics and the Health Services Manager," *Hospital & Health Services Administration 29* (March/April 1984): 120–136.

4. Robert M. Veatch, "Professional Ethics: New Principles for Physicians?" *Hastings Center Report 10* (June 1980): 17.

5. American Medical Association, "Principles of Ethics," 1980.

6. American Nurses Association, "Code for Nurses with Interpretative Statements," 1985, i.

7. Ibid., iii.

8. American Medical Association, "Principles of Ethics."

9. American College of Healthcare Executives, "Code of Ethics," 1988.

10. American Medical Association, "Principles of Ethics."

11. Darr, "Administrative Ethics."

12. Walter J. Wentz and Terence F. Moore, "Administrative Success: Key Ingredients," *Hospital & Health Services Administration* spec. 2 (1981): 85–93.

5

∞

ORGANIZATIONAL RESPONSES TO ETHICAL PROBLEMS

THUS FAR, LITTLE HAS BEEN said about the specific means used to analyze and solve administrative and biomedical ethical problems. For either type of problem, the starting points are the organization's philosophy and the manager's personal ethic. The philosophy establishes moral direction and a framework for the mission. The manager's personal ethic is crucial. In solving ethical problems, that ethic provides both the specificity and comprehensiveness the organizational philosophy may (but should not) lack. External constraints on the organization, such as criminal and civil laws and derivative regulations, set a minimum standard. For example, federal guidelines to protect human subjects of experimentation should serve as a starting point in developing the organization's independent relationship with patients who participate in research.

The primary established means for problem solving biomedical ethical issues are institutional review boards (IRBs) and institutional ethics committees (IECs). Although they provide limited assistance in solving administrative ethical problems, IRBs and IECs are useful in preventing or solving problems arising from biomedical ethical issues.

The manager is employed and personal and professional ethics are applied in the context of the organizational philosophy. Religious sisters who are managers are guided by the moral values of their religion. Managers in state and federal government must adhere to state or federal statutes prohibiting conflicts of interest. Many managers, however, are guided primarily by a personal ethic, as supplemented by the codes of their professional groups.

INSTITUTIONAL REVIEW BOARDS (IRBs)

IRBs are established to protect human subjects who participate in experimentation. IRBs are required by many federal agencies when they grant funds or regulate research. In the health services field, the Department of Health and Human Services (HHS) and the Food and Drug Administration (FDA) are the most important. Other federal agencies that require IRBs include the Environmental Protection Agency (EPA), the National Science Foundation (NSF), and the Consumer Product Safety Commission (CPSC).

Research funded wholly or in part through HHS that involves human subjects must be reviewed in a prescribed manner by an IRB that meets HHS criteria. Appendix C reproduces HHS's "Policy for Protection of Human Research Subjects." Two types of exceptions—exempt research and expedited review—are discussed later in this section.

FDA requirements are similar to those of HHS. Regardless of the source of funding, compliance with FDA guidelines, including the use of IRBs, is necessary if FDA approval for the drugs, biologicals, or medical devices under study is sought.

What other regulation of research exists? Virtually no states regulate research. Where no state regulation exists, the only source of formal control is the organization. Even where state regulation does exist, there are usually no controls on innovative treatments or on surgical intervention, including experimental surgery. In these situations, and in circumstances in which research is unregulated, the only control is that exercised by the organization through its managers and medical staff, or the researcher's personal ethic. Anecdotal evidence suggests that a physician who tries an old drug in new ways, or attempts a novel surgical procedure, will probably not be reviewed. It is thus imperative that the organization have effective procedures, especially quality assurance programs.

Membership and Purpose

Both HHS and FDA require that an IRB be competent to review research proposals for conformance with applicable law, standards of professional conduct and practice, and institutional commitment and regulations.[1] IRBs acceptable to HHS have a minimum of five members who are expected to have varying backgrounds (at least one member must have professional interests that are nonscientific) and who are capable of reviewing research proposals and activities of the type commonly performed by the organization.

The IRB acceptable to HHS must apply several requirements in reviewing research activities. These include:

- Minimizing risk to subjects
- Determining that risks are reasonable relative to anticipated benefits
- Selecting research subjects equitably
- Obtaining and documenting appropriate consent from research subjects or legally authorized representatives
- Monitoring data to ensure safety
- Protecting privacy and confidentiality
- Developing special protections when consent is obtained from persons likely to be vulnerable to coercion or undue influence, such as persons with acute or severe physical or mental illness, or persons who are economically or educationally disadvantaged

In addition, a number of special provisions identify the information needed for informed consent.

The FDA uses the same basic elements of consent as HHS, but has special provisions for situations in which the human subject is confronted with a life-threatening situation that necessitates use of the test article and in which the subject cannot give legally effective consent, for situations in which time is insufficient to obtain consent from the subject's legal representative, and for situations in which no alternative method of generally recognized therapy that provides an equal or greater likelihood of saving the subject's life is available.

New IRB Requirements

In 1981, new regulations eliminated a previous requirement that any HHS funding necessitated use of its guidelines in research that was not funded by HHS but that was performed in the same organization. This marked a major shift in the federal government's philosophy about its role in protecting human subjects and in research generally. The change places additional responsibilities on both managers and researchers, who must rely on their own moral integrity and personal ethic. In the long term, this change may cause states to become more involved in regulation and review of nonfederal research activities. A controversy in research activities, such as the Willowbrook case (detailed later in this section) will undoubtedly trigger a reaction by state health officials.

As a practical matter, organizations with multiple sources of funding, one of which is the federal government, will likely use the same IRB for all formal research activities. It is easy to slip, however, and managers must be alert to the potential for ethical problems in both formal research programs and isolated innovative therapy activities or surgical experimentation by members of the staff.

A mix of differing moral values is found in HHS regulations. The principle of beneficence and its subsidiary, cost–benefit analysis, is applied to determine the value of results expected from the research. Conversely, a clear Kantian (deontological) perspective and principles of respect for persons and nonmaleficence underlie the requirements for consent, privacy, and confidentiality.

Despite the emphasis on respect for persons and nonmaleficence, the regulations permit nontherapeutic research on children. A risk–benefit ratio is applied, and no child can be placed in unnecessary jeopardy. Because nontherapeutic research on children is condemned by some prominent commentators, however, very little of it is done.

Hepatitis for Children with Mental Retardation?

Willowbrook State Hospital was an institution for care of people with mental retardation. It was located in Staten Island, New York. When the story of Willowbrook was made public in 1971, it had over 5,000 residents.

Dr. Saul Krugman was a consultant in pediatrics and infectious diseases. When he began work at Willowbrook in the early 1950s, he discovered that major infectious diseases, including hepatitis, measles, shigellosis, parasitic infections, and respiratory infections, were prevalent. These conditions were similar to those at similar facilities elsewhere in the country. Dr. Krugman and his colleagues undertook a study of the diseases, including research on a measles vaccine and hepatitis.

In 1956, Dr. Krugman and Drs. Joan Giles and Jack Hammond began studies on hepatitis. In the final phase, the research involved 68 children aged 3–10 years during the period 1965–1970. The researchers injected an infected serum to produce hepatitis in the patient-subjects in their research unit. The objective was to gain a better understanding of hepatitis, and possibly develop methods of immunizing against it. The research was approved by the Armed Forces Epidemiological Board, one of the funders of the research; the executive faculty and the Committee on Human Experimentation of New York University, where Dr. Krugman held a faculty position; and the New York State Department of Mental Hygiene.

The researchers defended their decision to expose the children to strains of hepatitis on the following grounds:

1. The subjects were exposed to the same strains that existed naturally in the institution.
2. The subjects were admitted to a special, well-equipped, and well-staffed unit where they were isolated from exposure to other infectious diseases prevalent in the institution. The health risk to subjects was thus lower for those in the experiment than it was for those in the hospital at-large, where multiple infections occurred.
3. The subjects were likely to have a subclinical infection followed by immunity to the particular hepatitis virus.

Moreover, only those children whose parents gave informed consent participated in the experiment.[2]

Conditions at Willowbrook during the time of the research were deplorable, but similar to those at other facilities of the same type. Conditions were so bad that parents of patients were likely to prefer that their children be part of the research group—and thus purposely infected with hepatitis—than to have them live among the general population at Willowbrook. The research protocol was approved by prominent review bodies and the experiment continued for 16 years (from 1956–1971). A storm of adverse publicity resulted when the experimentation at Willowbrook was made public in 1967 by a New York state senator, who charged that children were being used as human guinea pigs. Despite this charge, the research continued. In 1971, the research produced spectacular results when Dr. Krugman and his colleagues were able to immunize a small group of children against serum hepatitis. These preliminary results were hailed as a major scientific breakthrough. In defending the research, Dr. Krugman reported that the injections to induce hepatitis in the research group were given only after great thought and professional discretion, and only with the informed consent of the parents. He stated that the doses were small and that inoculations usually produced the infections without making the children sick.

In 1975, a federal court ordered that Willowbrook reduce its patient load to 250 or fewer beds, and that patients be given the assistance needed to achieve their fullest potential. The order was to be met within 6 years. Complying with the order required major changes, including deinstitutionalization. By April 1982, progress had been made, but major goals remained unmet, and a federal court was successfully petitioned to appoint a special master to supervise the reform program. In January 1984, Governor Cuomo promised to close the facility, which still housed about 1,000 residents. The Willowbrook story continued when the federal government denied $22 million in Medicaid funds because of a chronic lack of adequate treatment and occupational therapy programs, and a finding on at least one occasion that there was not enough food for the patients. Living and bathing conditions—conditions not unlike those that had been identified 15 years earlier—were also found to be unsatisfactory. Willowbrook closed at the end of 1987, after a federal court approved a final settlement.

The presence of an IRB and federal guidelines would not necessarily have prevented research such as that that went on at Willowbrook from going forward. Federal guidelines allow nontherapeutic research on children, provided consent is given by those legally able to do so. An IRB applying only federal guidelines thus could have approved this research. The organizational philosophy could, however, apply a more demanding standard—one prohibiting research on children.

For Willowbrook and similar institutions, the horrific conditions should have caused a reconsideration of whether to allow them to continue to function—a question of justice in allocating state funds (macroallocation). Absent that, however, the principles of respect for persons, beneficence, and nonmaleficence should have been applied within the context of the situation. Dr. Krugman and his colleagues make a convincing case for undertaking and continuing the research.

Exempt Research and Expedited Review

The 1981 HHS regulations identified exempt research and research warranting expedited review as two new categories to which different provisions apply. Exempt research includes primarily research in the behavioral sciences. It includes certain educational practices and testing, interview procedures and observation, and collection of already available data. Examples include: research conducted in an established or commonly accepted educational setting involving normal educational practices, use of educational tests if information from these sources maintains the subjects' anonymity, and observing public behavior (e.g., collecting or studying existing data and records) if certain safeguards are met. Expedited review applies special procedures for research in which no more than minimal risk is involved and in which human subjects have very limited involvement. Examples include: collection of hair and nail clippings in a nondisfiguring manner; collection of deciduous teeth; use of voice recordings; study of existing data, documents, records, and pathological or diagnostic specimens; and moderate exercise by volunteers. These changes greatly facilitate several kinds of research.

INSTITUTIONAL ETHICS COMMITTEES (IECs)

This section recommends that complex health services organizations, especially acute care hospitals, have an ethics committee with at least two subcommittees, each of which addresses different types of ethical issues. (An alternative is to have an ethics committee for administrative issues and an ethics committee for biomedical ethical issues.) Specializing in this fashion is necessary because a committee able to grapple with matters of biomedical ethics is unlikely to be well prepared to solve problems of administrative ethics. Further specialization may be needed within the two broad categories of administrative and biomedical ethics. For example, it may be necessary to set up an infant care review committee. Care must be taken that committee proliferation does not cause inefficient overlap, however. Because of the need to solve general, organizationwide issues and specific, perhaps very technical, problems, the committee with subcommittees model may be most effective.

Concern about the activities of ethics committees is sounded by Veatch, who suggests three models: 1) an autonomy model that implements decisions of competent patients whose wishes are known; 2) a social justice model to grapple with broad issues such as organizational health care policy, resource allocation, cost effectiveness, and the like; and 3) a patient benefit model to make decisions for patients unable to make decisions for themselves.[3] He argues that in many respects, these roles are mutually exclusive, because different ethical tasks emphasize different ethical principles. Ethics committees using an autonomy model are accountable to the patient, whereas ethics committees concerned with social justice must be accountable to the organization. Veatch's concern is shared by other experts in the field. In a committee, organizational concerns can easily overwhelm concerns about patient goals.[4] Furthermore, values of committee members might differ from those of patients. Of the three models developed by Veatch, the first and the third emphasize biomedical ethical issues. The second could address administrative, as well as biomedical issues, if it were determined desirable to mix the two in one committee.

Before considering ethical problems within the organization, IECs must develop a statement of their ethic. This is not a determination of how to solve each problem, but a statement of general principles intended to guide deliberations and decision making. The overall framework for that ethic is provided by the organizational philosophy and mission. Only by undertaking and successfully concluding such deliberations can IECs be effective. This exercise should also be useful in identifying and minimizing differences in members' personal ethics.

As initially conceived by the court in the Karen Ann Quinlan case, IECs had a very limited scope. These committees were no more than prognosis committees that assisted in answering questions about the terminally ill, especially about whether to continue life support. In some organizations, IECs with this role are called "God squads" since they determine when life support is to be withdrawn and the patient declared dead. IECs should have and typically do have a much broader role.

An early source of information about the structure, procedures, activities, and effectiveness of IECs used in solving biomedical ethical issues was a national survey done for the President's Commission, the results of which were published in 1983.[5] No hospital with fewer than 200 beds was found to have an IEC, and even in large hospitals IECs were not ubiquitous. Larger hospitals, particularly those with teaching programs, were most likely to have an IEC. The study estimated that there were fewer than 100 IECs in U.S. hospitals. The Quinlan decision seems to have been crucial in motivating some hospitals to establish IECs: in New Jersey, where they were most common, 71% had been formed as a result of that case.

Surveys in 1983 and 1985 by the National Society of Patient Representatives showed rapid growth in IECs. In 1983, 26% of hospitals responding to the survey had IECs. This figure rose to 59% in 1985. Many committees were established in response to the Baby Doe controversy, as hospitals developed internal processes to solve ethical issues. Since then, IECs have broadened their roles, and have undertaken tasks such as developing do-not-resuscitate (DNR) and patient consent policies, advising on withholding or withdrawing life support, and educational programs.[6] The methodology used in the surveys caused disproportionate numbers of large hospitals to respond. Thus, caution must be used in generalizing the findings. The findings on rapid growth are consistent with the research by the American Academy of Pediatrics reported below. The findings of a telephone survey show little recent growth in the number of IECs, however.[7] It has been suggested that ethics committees have matured and it is time for them to reconsider their roles and determine whether they should be involved in new ways and in other aspects of the organization's activities.[8]

Membership

Results of the President's Commission study, shown in Table 1, suggest that biomedical IECs are interdisciplinary. Not surprisingly, physicians are the most

Table 1.   Biomedical institutional ethics committee membership

Member category	Median number of members per committee	Number (and percent) of committees reporting at least one member in this category
Physician	5.25	17 (100)
Clergy	1.05	14 (82)
Administrator	.58	9 (53)
Nurse	.44	8 (47)
Attorney	.35	7 (41)
Social worker	.21	5 (29)
Layperson	.15	4 (24)
House officer	.07	2 (12)
Other	.07	2 (12)

From President's Commission for the Study of Ethical Problems in Medicine and Biomedical and Behavioral Research. (1983). *Deciding to forego life-sustaining treatment: Ethical, medical, and legal issues in treatment decisions,* p. 450. Washington, DC: Government Printing Office.

common type of member, with an average of 5.25 physicians serving per committee. On average, every committee had at least one clergyman. Other professionals found on fewer than half the committees were attorneys, laypersons, social workers, and physicians in graduate education programs. Administrators are included far less frequently than physicians, and serve on only about half the committees. The commission did not find a strong community link, something that governing body members and individuals from the organization's service area can provide. Such persons bring an important perspective to decision making.[9] Managers, too, are underrepresented. This may reflect too little interest in clinical matters, generally—a problem managers must act to remedy.

An administrative IEC will have fewer clinical personnel and more representatives from the governing body and management. Clinical personnel must be included, however, since it is reasonable to conclude that research suggesting that organizations are most effective when they involve clinicians in management decision making also applies to solving problems of administrative ethics.

Purposes and Roles

IECs should undertake two roles of general importance to the organization and its staff. One is to develop or assist in developing the organizational philosophy and policies on ethical issues. The experience and range of its interdisciplinary membership is likely to assist in producing better reasoned and more thorough results. Education is the second role. The composition of the IEC and the experience of its members make it a natural reservoir of knowledge and expertise.

These resources should be available to the governing body and staff. Such attributes add sophistication and will improve the quality of clinical and administrative decision making.

In terms of biomedical ethics, major benefits of IECs reported in the President's Commission study include facilitating decision making by: clarifying important issues, shaping consistent hospital policies about life support, and providing opportunities for professionals to air disagreements. The committees were not found to be particularly effective at increasing the ability of patients' families to influence decisions or at educating professionals about issues relevant to life support decisions. The purposes of the committees, reported in Table 2, show that the commission found IECs to be directed at solving biomedical ethical problems.

The study also reported two general observations:

1. . . . committees that do exist are not involved in large numbers of cases. Existing committees reviewed an average of only one case per year.
2. The composition and function of committees identified in the survey would

Table 2. Purposes of biomedical institutional ethics committees

Purpose	Percent classifying this as a stated purpose	Percent classifying this as an actual function
Provide counsel and support to physicians	59 (10)	69 (11)
Make ethical/social policy for care of critically ill	47 (8)	38 (6)
Review ethical issues in patient care decisions	53 (9)	56 (9)
Provide counsel and support to other professionals	35 (6)	31 (5)
Determine medical prognosis	29 (5)	25 (4)
Provide counsel and support to patients and families	29 (5)	31 (5)
Make final decisions about life support	13 (3)	31 (5)
Determine continuing education needs	18 (3)	19 (3)
Other	12 (2)	12 (2)

Note: Numbers in parentheses refer to frequency of response.

From President's Commission for the Study of Ethical Problems in Medicine and Biomedical and Behavioral Research. (1983). *Deciding to forego life-sustaining treatment: Ethical, medical, and legal issues in treatment decisions,* p. 451. Washington, DC: Government Printing Office.

not allay many of the concerns of patients' rights advocates about patient representation and control. Committees were clearly dominated by physicians and other health professionals. The majority of committees did not allow patients to attend or request meetings, although family members were more often permitted to do so. Yet, chairmen generally regarded their committees as effective.[10]

This latter finding suggests that health services managers should be particularly alert to patient autonomy—a matter affecting several aspects of the organization, but especially resource allocation and consent. Anecdotal evidence suggests that these findings of the President's Commission are for the most part true today.

Relationships

The IEC's relationships vary depending on its specific role. There are general and specific levels of activity. General levels of activity are organizationwide, and can be divided into biomedical and administrative ethics. Examples include reconsidering the organizational philosophy, developing a conflict of interest policy, or guiding macroallocation decisions. Specific levels of activity are individual cases in which ethical questions arise. Examples include determining whether a particular activity is consistent with the organizational philosophy or whether a conflict exists.

The IEC should be proactive in developing and revising the organizational philosophy and in considering the ethical implications of macro resource allocation questions. Similarly, it should take the initiative in reviewing and revising the consent process. However, it may choose a more passive role, and wait to be consulted in specific instances of conflicts of interest and misuse of confidential information (in the case of an administrative IEC) or for specific clinical matters (in the case of a biomedical IEC).

There is evidence from the President's Commission study that IECs involved in biomedical ethics problem solving are most effective when they wait to be consulted rather than interpose themselves. A consultative role means committees make recommendations, not final decisions.[11] IEC participation in biomedical and administrative decision making may be optional or mandatory. Following advice given by an IEC could also be made optional or mandatory. The combinations are shown in Table 3.

Physicians are unlikely to accept mandatory-mandatory involvement by a biomedical IEC. Furthermore, this may not be desirable in the majority of situations, where a competent physician is willing to develop alternatives and communicate them effectively to the patient and other concerned persons. Even where the physician is unwilling to share decision making with the members of an ethics committee, however, there are benefits to having advice available.

An important aspect of organizing an IEC is the question of where it should reside administratively. This issue was not addressed by the President's Commission study. Options include making the IEC a standing committee of

Table 3.   Matrix of possible roles for IECs

Involvement of committee in decision making	Acceptance and use of advice given by IEC
Optional	Optional
Optional	Mandatory
Mandatory	Optional
Mandatory	Mandatory

the board, of the medical staff, or of the administration. The fear that the IEC will be dominated by physicians has led some experts to suggest that it be a board or administration committee. Similarly, no committee member should represent only one specific interest or group.[12]

INFANT CARE REVIEW COMMITTEES (ICRCs)

Federal legislation enacted in 1984 directs HHS to encourage establishment of infant care review committees (ICRCs) within health services facilities, especially facilities with tertiary level neonatal care units. ICRCs are specialized IECs that focus on the biomedical ethical problems of infants with life-threatening conditions. In the guidelines developed by HHS, ICRCs are ethics committees that provide information and education, recommend institutional policies and guidelines, and offer counsel and review of issues related to infant care. The guidelines make it clear that HHS considers it prudent to establish an ICRC, but that the organization makes the final decision. The background to these regulations is provided in Chapter 10.

Certain aspects of membership in and administration of ICRCs recommended in the guidelines are notable. Membership should include persons from varied disciplines and perspectives, because a multidisciplinary approach provides expertise to supply and evaluate all pertinent information. The committee should be large enough to represent diverse viewpoints, but not so large as to hinder effectiveness. Recommended membership includes a practicing physician (e.g., pediatrician, neonatologist, pediatric surgeon), practicing nurse, hospital administrator, social worker, representative of a disability group, lay community member, and a member of the facility's medical staff, who serves as chairman.[13] The recommendation that there be a representative of a disability group is counter to the principle that specific groups not have representatives.

HHS recommends that the ICRC have adequate staff support, including legal counsel; that it recommend procedures to ensure that both hospital personnel and patient families are fully informed of its existence, functions, and 24-hour availability; that it inform itself of pertinent legal requirements and procedures, including state law requiring reports of known or suspected medical neglect; and that it maintain records of deliberations and summary descriptions of the cases considered and their disposition.[14]

HHS's recommended form and activities for ICRCs are similar to those reported in a 1984 study of 710 hospitals with special care pediatric units. The American Academy of Pediatrics (AAP) found that of the 426 respondents, 56.5% had ICRCs or IECs. Three quarters of hospitals without such a committee were considering establishing one. The remaining 25% handle ethical problems by other means, including waiting for clarification of legal issues and acting on that information, or using a university committee or state board. The committee activity mentioned most frequently was consultation on difficult ethical decisions. This was followed by advising parents, advising physicians (when consulted), and educating staff. Developing hospital policies was rated as the third most important function of an ICRC. The composition of the committee was similar to that found by the President's Commission study.[15]

The percentage of hospitals with ethics committees reported in the AAP study is much higher than that found in the study by the President's Commission. The AAP findings are consistent with the findings of the National Society of Patient Representatives. The Commission's research was done several years before the AAP study, and differences in findings suggest a major change in the interim, at least regarding numbers of ICRCs. In fact, the AAP report commented that there was evidence that many committees had been formed recently. The AAP report found that more administrators were serving on ICRCs than had been found to serve on IECs in the earlier President's Commission study. Greater involvement of managerial staff in biomedical ethical decision making is very desirable.

SPECIALIZED PERSONNEL

Ethics Consultation Services (ECSs)

One way in which health services organizations provide specialized personnel to advise and assist in solving biomedical ethics problems is to establish an ethics consultation service (ECS). Doing so is very much like establishing a clinical service. The ECS is staffed by ethicists, who have graduate degrees in philosophy, often at the doctoral level, and clinical personnel, who may be physicians or other caregivers. The clinicians have a special interest and/or preparation in ethics, and provide an effective bridge between the ethicist and the clinical staff attending the patient. They serve, too, as a resource to the ethicists. In this model, an ethicist is on call and the clinical member of the ECS is involved as needed. The ECS reports to the IEC, and the IEC develops and recommends policy to the governing body. The IEC also serves as a sounding board for problems that develop during ethics consultation. A variant of this approach has a primary consultant who is assisted by other participating members of the ECS. Both the primary consultants and those assisting have a variety of backgrounds, but they all have intensive and specialized training in ethics, and participate in case reviews, ethics instruction, and regular meetings of the ECS staff.[16]

Ethicists

A less formal approach is commonly found in larger hospitals. Its concept need not be and should not be limited to them, however. These hospitals often have ethicists on their staffs, either full time or part time. As in the case of ECSs, these ethicists are often philosophers with Ph.D.s, who may be members of the faculty at a university or medical school and who consult with clinical staff on biomedical ethical issues. Organizations that want the assistance of an ethicist should not limit their search to universities or medical schools, but should consider anyone with specialized preparation in ethics and its application in the health field. Here, as in the case of the ECS, the ethicist is the clinically oriented, problem-solving extension of an IEC.

DISPUTE RESOLUTION

The American Arbitration Association (AAA) has conducted seminars to train hospice organization professionals to resolve disputes over appropriate patient care more effectively.[17] This need to resolve disputes is necessary because various health care professionals have different views about issues and consequently about cases. The objective of improved dispute resolution is to weld a multidisciplinary group into a cohesive and mutually supportive team so that they can resolve their differences and maintain the quality of patient care. Such formal preparation could assist IECs, ICRCs, as well as IRBs. It is overly optimistic to assume that the mere act of establishing an interdisciplinary ethics committee means that it will be successful. Specific preparation in resolving disputes is a way to improve its effectiveness.

ASSISTANCE FOR MANAGERS

This discussion has described means to assist the organization and its administrative and clinical staffs in solving administrative and biomedical ethical problems. Analogues to IRBs and IECs available to assist managers in identifying and solving administrative ethical problems are not as well developed, but with patience and perseverance they can be.

Despite the lack of formal mechanisms, managers and organizations have developed de facto means to identify and solve administrative ethical problems. These include adopting specific policies (discussed in Chapter 6) and establishing management committees and task forces, both of which increasingly include physicians. There are also guidelines developed by professional associations. Of course, the manager's personal ethic and the organization's philosophy continue to be major sources of guidance.

The Administrative IEC

The CEO of Community Health Plan had been approached by a group from "north of the river." This area of the city was economically depressed, and had lost many of its health services delivery organizations and physicians to the suburbs over the previous decade. It seemed to be in a downward vortex with no apparent end. Decreasing numbers of insured patients meant that organizations were less and less able to continue serving the area. The city-owned hospital had made several ill-fated attempts to serve the area north of the river with a clinic system, but its efforts had been scandal ridden. The system was a political football with little credibility in the community.

The representatives from north of the river were community leaders, none of whom appeared to have political ambitions. They seemed genuinely willing to do whatever they could to assist in securing high-quality health services for the community. They proposed that Community Health Plan establish and staff three storefront clinics in the area. The community leaders stated they would get volunteers to remodel the facilities and work in clerical capacities.

The CEO was describing the proposed activity to the administrative IEC, which included members of the governing board, managers, and physicians and other caregivers. In making the presentation, the CEO stressed the plan's historical role in providing health services to those in need, its not-for-profit status, and its continuing modest surplus. The members listened patiently, but the minute the CEO was finished all of them seemed to speak at once.

Several were opposed and made the following points about the suggested venture:

1. The area north of the river was the city's responsibility. Providing care to the needy was not something a small, not-for-profit health plan should attempt.
2. The organization's primary obligation was to enhance benefits for their enrollees, not to get involved in new schemes. New services had been requested by several of their physicians and many plan members.
3. The modest surplus the plan had accumulated over several years could easily be consumed by the proposed venture. The chief financial officer noted they were expecting an increase in reinsurance premiums in the next quarter.
4. If the plan pulled the city's political chestnuts out of the fire by providing even stopgap assistance, the city would never

get its house in order and develop the system needed north of the river.

Several spoke in favor of working north of the river:

1. Helping the north of the river community was the right thing to do. The people there deserved health services. It was noted that their own start had come about when several physicians in the community had fought the prevailing attitude among their peers about prepaid practice.
2. Those opposed were putting dollars ahead of people's health. They must be willing to assist those less fortunate.
3. Plan members would support such an initiative if it were properly explained to them.
4. The positive publicity would further the plan's interests by increasing the number of enrollees.

It seemed to the CEO this was a no-win situation. The organizational philosophy was not well developed, and the proposal was a major step. Something should be done to assist the north of the river community. The IEC members were raising valid points that merited further discussion.

This case identifies the dilemmas arising from macroallocation decisions about resources. The complexity is particularly great here because the plan is being asked to volunteer assistance and to do so from its own meager surplus. Theories of justice in allocating resources relevant to the case include: retribution, or compensatory justice (distribution of resources in a manner that makes up for past wrongs); just deserts (help would go to those who have not earned it and the plan's leadership has no right to risk the plan's solvency, which is something the membership paid to achieve); egalitarianism in access to health services and whether it is government's responsibility to provide it to the community north of the river; and utility as a prospectively determined element of beneficence. A major problem for the health plan is that it has not considered this aspect of its relationship with special subsets of the community in its organizational philosophy and subsidiary mission statement. It would do well to develop this role prospectively in a comprehensive fashion, rather than address it on an ad hoc basis.

CONCLUSION

Decision-making and operational activities of all health services organizations raise ethical considerations. In this regard, two challenges confront the manager. The first is to recognize the presence of ethical problems. The second is to apply analytical and reasoning processes that solve these issues, thereby enhancing the quality of decision making. Applied ethics is a newly emerging aspect of health services management. Its effective use enhances the very purpose for which the organization exists.

Economic pressures because of cost cutting by third-party payors—especially the federal government—and new competitive pressures will affect all health services organizations, especially acute care hospitals. Managers may be tempted to use economic justifications for decisions that implicitly, or even explicitly, affect quality of care negatively. The potential for conflict between economic interests and quality considerations lies not far below the surface in most relationships with patients. The technical nature of health services and the inability of average consumers to judge results make it imperative that all persons associated with delivery expend every effort to further the quality of care and protect the interests of patients.

ECSs and ethicists can be involved on a more discretionary basis to assist in identifying and analyzing the moral obligations, rights, responsibilities, and considerations of justice that bear on a general issue, or on the ethical issues in a specific clinical case.[18] The literature suggests that they can assist physicians, and are more likely to be used than are biomedical ethics committees, which are seen by physicians as cost ineffective. Beyond considerations of efficiency, it may be more palatable for physicians to consult with a single ethicist than to seek guidance from a committee. Ethicists can serve a similar function for managers by assisting them in identifying and solving administrative ethics problems and working with an administrative IEC.

IECs tend to be limited to solving the more complex questions, some of which may come under mandatory review (e.g., organizational philosophy). This chapter has focused on IECs in hospitals. Committees have the potential to provide assistance in a wide range of health services organizations, including nursing facilities (NFs), health maintenance organizations (HMOs), and hospices. Such organizations face many of the same ethical problems faced by hospitals. Hospices and nursing facilities, for example, face issues related to death and dying. HMOs face issues related to resource allocation and physician incentive plans.

Codes of ethics can point managers in the right direction, but managers must develop and be guided by a personal ethic—one that focuses on their independent duty to the patient.

NOTES

1. President's Commission for the Study of Ethical Problems in Medicine and Biomedical and Behavioral Research, *Protecting Human Subjects,* Appendix B (Washington, DC: Government Printing Office, 1981).

2. Articles from several issues of the *New York Times* were used in preparing the Willowbrook case and the background information, including: January 11, 12, and 13, 1967; March 24, 1971; April 18, 1971; January 11, 1972; May 25, 1981; January 8, 1984; April 19, 1985; and March 3, 1987.

3. Robert M. Veatch, "Ethics Committees Proliferation in Hospitals Predicted," *Hospitals 57,* no. 13, (July 1983): 48–49.

4. Marilyn M. Mannisto, "Orchestrating an Ethics Committee: Who Should Be on It, Where Does It Best Fit?" *Trustee 38,* no. 4 (April 1985): 17–20.

5. President's Commission for the Study of Ethical Problems in Medicine and Biomedical and Behavioral Research, *Deciding to Forego Life-Sustaining Treatment: Ethical, Medical, and Legal Issues in Treatment Decisions* (Washington, DC: Government Printing Office, 1983), 443.

6. American Hospital Association, "New Survey Shows Rapid Growth in Hospital Ethics Committees," Press release, September 1, 1985.

7. "Right-to Die: An Executive Report," *Hospitals* (November 20, 1989): 34.

8. Cynthia B. Cohen, ed., "Ethics Committees," *Hastings Center Report 20* (March/April 1990): 29–34.

9. Mannisto, "Orchestrating," 18–19.

10. President's Commission, *Human Subjects,* 443.

11. Benjamin Freedman, "One Philosopher's Experience on an Ethics Committee," *Hastings Center Report 11* (April 1981): 20–22.

12. Mannisto, "Orchestrating," 18–19.

13. Department of Health and Human Services, Office of Human Development Services, "Services and Treatment for Disabled Infants; Model Guidelines for Health Care Providers to Establish Infant Care Review Committees," *Federal Register 50,* no. 72 (April 15, 1985): 14893.

14. Ibid.

15. "Summary: Survey of Infant Care Review Committees." Paper delivered at the Annual Meeting of the American Academy of Pediatrics, Chicago, Illinois, September 18, 1984.

16. John C. Fletcher, Margo L. White, and Philip J. Foubert, "Biomedical Ethics and an Ethics Consultation Service at the University of Virginia," *HEC Forum 2,* no. 2 (1990): 89–99.

17. "Arbitration Times," American Arbitration Association (Summer 1984): 7.

18. John C. Fletcher, Norman Quist, and Albert R. Jonsen, *Ethics Consultation in Health Care* (Ann Arbor: Health Administration Press, 1989).

III

∞

ADMINISTRATIVE ETHICAL ISSUES

WITH FEW EXCEPTIONS, there are ethical dimensions to all of the administrative problems that arise in managing health services organizations and programs. Ethical problems in health services are qualitatively different from ethical problems in the business world.

The literature on business ethics burgeoned in the 1980s, and courses in business policy and ethics are now common in graduate and undergraduate business programs. There is, however, little tradition in business of an independent duty or obligation beyond that established by law—the emphasis in business has been and is on profitability and *caveat emptor.* The business ethics literature discusses concepts such as honesty, integrity, benevolence, the duties employees have toward each other and toward the organization, and the duties organizations have toward employees. Here there is some similarity with health services. Lacking, however, is the concept of respect for persons, with its emphasis on autonomy, fidelity, and confidentiality. Nor is beneficence a focus in business ethics. The principle of justice is found only at the periphery of business ethics. These differences betweeen business and health services are cited here not as a criticism of the business world, but to distinguish the two fields of endeavor, whose foci and purposes are simply different.

The view of both the public and the health services sector itself has been that there is a higher calling in health services—one that goes well beyond the bottom line. Codes of ethics are important in defining this calling and the duty of managers. Much of this definition stems from the link with physicians, as well as from the not-for-profit status common in many health services organizations. In the case of acute care hospitals, the historic link with religious orders and humanistic motivation has created a special image. In total, this has resulted in a strong emphasis on the caring, as well as the curing, aspect of health services delivery. It strongly reflects the societal view that the sick are a unique group—one with special status—who need protection and are not to be exploited.

The issues of administrative ethics confronting the health services manager run the gamut from conflict of interest to governing body and medical staff relations to duty toward the patient. Although they can be subtle and appear in many guises, these problems are identifiable and solvable to alert and conscientious managers.

In this part of the book, administrative ethical issues are identified and discussed. These are very different from the biomedical ethical issues considered in Part IV. (Although the distinction between administrative and biomedical ethical issues is important, it is often blurred in practice. The best example of this is the issue of consent.) A major difference between administrative and biomedical ethical issues is that administrative ethics are less likely to affect individual patients directly, but rather will primarily affect the manager's relationship with the organization, peers, profession, and, perhaps, the community. Biomedical ethics almost always affect individuals or specific groups, but there are exceptions, such as issues of resource allocation, that may affect both macro- and microallocation. This is not to say that each type of ethical problem does not have an actual or potential effect on the other. The primary focus of each type of problem is usually different, however.

6

∞

CONFLICTS OF INTEREST AND FIDUCIARY DUTY

CONFLICT OF INTEREST IS THE MOST often reported administrative ethical problem confronting health services organizations. The American College of Healthcare Executives (ACHE) Code devotes more attention to conflict of interest than to any other ethical problem. Trade associations, such as the American Hospital Association (AHA), have issued policy statements about conflicts of interest. A conflict of interest occurs when a person owes duties to two or more persons or organizations and meeting a duty to one of them causes derogation of a duty to another. The classic case arises when a decision maker—a director (trustee) or a manager—is also a director of a corporation with which the health services organization does business. The manager's duties to both sides makes it impossible for decisions on matters affecting both to be objective. Similar conflicts arise for clinicians, too. Conflicts between duties owed different patients by the same physicians are an important reason, for example, to separate the organ transplant team from physicians treating the potential donor. Other conflicts of interest occur when duties owed the organization by a physician are in conflict with those owed patients or colleagues, or when similarly diagnosed patients in different payment categories are provided different care in the same organization or by the same physician.

Conflict of interest is an insidious problem into which one can slip almost without realizing what is happening. The ACHE Code notes that the line between acceptable and unacceptable behavior is sometimes fine. This pragmatic view recognizes that normal business interaction frequently establishes relationships that, if carried too far, result in a conflict of interests.

The manager's relationships with the organization and interactions with the health system and other organizations in it can cause conflicts of interest to occur. In addition to potentially affecting the manager's relationship with the organization, conflicts of interest can affect managers' relationships with the profession and their personal development.

Conflicts of interest can be very subtle, and can affect all managerial activities. Has the manager who uses a position of influence and power to gain titles, stature, and income at the expense of patient care acted ethically? Is the manager who is lax in developing and implementing an effective patient consent policy and process acting ethically? Is it ethical for a manager to insist on reviewing all reports and information for the governing body and to demand that reports on the competence of the administrative staff be prepared and presented in the best light? Is it ethical for a manager who believes problems may exist in the department of surgery to do nothing to prove or disprove their presence? Is it ethical for managers who have serious concerns about their abilities to continue managing? An element of complexity is added to these questions because many ethical problems have legal implications. In any case, managers must view themselves as having an independent, positive duty toward the patient.

Managers must avoid any hint of wrongdoing, especially the suggestion of divided loyalties. When a hospital CEO owns stock in a corporation that does the hospital's data processing, and the principal stockholder and CEO of the data-processing corporation is also the hospital comptroller, the whole arrangement has a bad odor. This odor is present regardless of the price or other advantages the hospital obtains. Observers are likely to think the transaction has hidden flaws that are detrimental to the organization or its patients, and that the managers are reaping a personal advantage. Attempts to convince the public otherwise probably reinforce the perception of wrongdoing. The only course of action is to avoid arrangements or entanglements that have any hint of conflicts of interests. The problem is put well by Harlan Cleveland in *The Future Executive*. "If this action is held up to public scrutiny, will I still feel that it is what I should have done, and how I should have done it?"[1]

FIDUCIARY DUTY

Fiduciary is an ethical and legal concept arising from Roman jurisprudence. A fiduciary relationship exists whenever confidence and trust on one side result in superiority and influence on the other. The presence of this superiority and influence raises duties of loyalty and responsibility. This broad definition suggests the presence of numerous fiduciary relationships in health services. Governing body members, for example, are fiduciaries. The duty of loyalty prevents them from using their position for personal gain, and they must act only in the organization's best interests. This has been interpreted to mean that no secret profits can be made in dealings with the organization, and that the member may not accept bribes or compete with the organization. The duty of responsibility requires governing body members to exercise reasonable care, skill, and diligence, as demanded by the circumstances.[2] Members of governing bodies have a duty to avoid both errors of omission and errors of commission. Breaching these duties could result in personal liability, whether the corporation is organized for profit or not.

Trusts are common in the health services field. Many not-for-profit health services organizations engaging in charitable activities were established because of a gift or bequest, and trustees are named to manage the trust's assets. Examples are trusts to defray the costs of a nursing unit or a specific clinical activity in a general acute care hospital. Other uses include funding schools of nursing or providing scholarships to educate health services personnel.

The term *trustee* is often used to describe governing body members of any not-for-profit corporation in the health services field, even though no trust is involved and they are not true trustees. Technically, the legally correct term for such people is *director* or *corporate director.* The term *trustee* seems to be preferred in the not-for-profit sector, however. This may be because directors of not-for-profit organizations want to be distinguished from governing body members in for-profit organizations, where the title director is used.

The legal standard for true trustees is much more stringent than that applied to directors of corporations or to persons who are responsible for monies or properties that are not held in trust. True trustees actually hold title to property or the corpus of the trust, and manage it for the beneficiary. The true trustee must act in good faith, and have undivided loyalty in administering the trust. All situations and relations that interfere with discharging these duties must be avoided. Breaching these standards results in personal liability. In many jurisdictions, the standard of care required of directors of not-for-profit corporations who are not true trustees is higher than that required of other corporate directors. The usual standard for directors who are not true trustees is that they are liable for ordinary negligence—mistakes in judgment. The minority rule is that directors must have committed gross negligence, typically defined as an intentional failure to perform a manifest duty in reckless disregard of the consequences, in order to be legally liable.

Sibley Hospital

An important court case involving governing body members of a health services organization is *Stern et al. v. Lucy Webb Hayes National Training School of Deaconesses and Missionaries et al.*[3] Sibley Hospital, a not-for-profit hospital in Washington, D.C. run by the Lucy Webb Hayes School, had a board of directors, whom it called "trustees," although they were not true trustees. David M. Stern sued Sibley on behalf of his minor son and other patients as a class. The complaint alleged that patients at Sibley Hospital had paid too much for care because several members of the board had engaged in mismanagement, nonmanagement, and self-dealing (succumbing to self-interest). It alleged further that these acts of omission and commission resulted from a conspiracy between those "trustees" and various financial institutions with which several were affiliated. The court found no evidence of a conspiracy. However, in considering the other allegations, it determined:

> The charitable corporation is a relatively new legal entity which does not fit neatly into the established common law categories of corporation and trust . . . the mod-

ern trend is to apply corporate rather than trust principles in determining the liability of the directors of a charitable corporation, because their functions are virtually indistinguishable from those of their "pure" corporate counterparts.[4]

This ruling held the defendant "trustees" to a less stringent standard of care.

The court found that the "trustees" had violated their duties as fiduciaries, even when held to the lesser standard. Mismanagement occurred because "trustees" ignored the investment sections of yearly audits, failed to acquire enough information to vote intelligently on opening new bank accounts, and generally failed to exercise even cursory supervision over hospital funds. Nonmanagement was evidenced by the same failure to exercise supervision, and was most starkly shown because even though certain "trustees" were repeatedly elected to the investment committee, they did not object when the committee failed to meet in over 10 years. The allegation of self-dealing was substantiated by several facts: a number of "trustees" were officers of banks in which the hospital kept hundreds of thousands of dollars in noninterest-bearing checking accounts, interest-bearing accounts paid less than market conditions would have permitted, and one "trustee" advised approval and voted to approve a contract for investment services with a corporation of which he was president.

The court did not find evidence of personal gain by the "trustees," although in several instances they had been associated with organizations that had benefited from the transactions. The absence of a conspiracy seems to have been significant in the ruling.

The court did not order any "trustees" removed from the board and no personal liability resulted from their wrongdoing. To prevent similar situations from happening in the future, the court ordered the board to: adopt a written investment policy, review its relevant committees to determine if all hospital assets conformed to the policy, and establish a regular process of disclosure of board members' business affiliations. In the meantime, the board had adopted guidelines on conflicts of interest recommended by the American Hospital Association (AHA). This action was long after the fact, but it demonstrated the board's good faith.

The current conflict of interest statement suggested by the AHA is shown in Figure 6. It reflects the corporate director standard, which is the less stringent standard.

The decision in the *Sibley* case was handed down in a trial court, not an appeals court, and therefore has limited legal significance as a precedent. Nonetheless, it is one of few cases that considers the standard of care for governing body members (directors) of not-for-profit organizations. Fiduciary duty requires governing body members to exercise reasonable care, skill, and diligence; under a negligence theory, they are liable for acts of commission or omission that violate this standard. Reasonable care means the care an ordinary, prudent director would exercise under the same or similar circumstances. The

Disclosure of certain interests of governing board members

WHEREAS, The proper governance of the nation's health care institutions depends on governing board members who give of their time for the benefit of their health communities, and,

WHEREAS, The giving of this service, because of the varied interests and backgrounds of the governing board members, may result in situations involving a dual interest that might be interpreted as conflict of interest, and,

WHEREAS, This service should not be rendered impossible solely by reason of duality of interest or possible conflict of interest; and,

WHEREAS, This service nevertheless carries with it a requirement of loyalty and fidelity to the institution served, it being the responsibility of the members of the board to govern the institution's affairs honestly and economically, exercising their best care, skill, and judgment for the benefit of the institution; and

WHEREAS, The matter of any duality of interest or possible conflict of interest can best be handled through full disclosure of any such interest, together with noninvolvement in any vote wherein the interest is involved:

NOW, THEREFORE, BE IT RESOLVED: That the following policy of duality and conflict of interest is hereby adopted:

1. Any duality of interest or possible conflict of interest on the part of any governing board member should be disclosed to the other members of the board and made a matter of record, either through an annual procedure or when the interest becomes a matter of board action.

2. Any governing board member having a duality of interest or possible conflict of interest on any matter should not vote or use his personal influence on the matter, and he should not be counted in determining the quorum for the meeting, even where permitted by law. The minutes of the meeting should reflect that a disclosure was made, the abstention from voting, and the quorum situation.

3. The foregoing requirements should not be construed as preventing the governing board member from briefly stating his position in the matter, nor from answering pertinent questions of other board members since his knowledge may be of great assistance.

BE IT FURTHER RESOLVED: That this policy be reviewed annually for the information and guidance of governing board members, and that any new member be advised of the policy upon entering on the duties of his office.

Figure 6. Confict of interest statement of the American Hospital Association (AHA). (Reprinted with permission from Resolution of Conflicts of Interest in Health Care Institutions, © 1975 by the American Hospital Association.)

rule enunciated by the court in *Sibley* is that governing body members (directors) of a not-for-profit corporation may be held liable for ordinary negligence, not only for gross negligence or willful misconduct. This is the same standard as that usually imposed on a director of a business enterprise.

CEOs and other managers are not fiduciaries in the same sense that directors are, but are held to a similarly defined standard—a duty to exercise reasonable care, skill, and diligence, or the care that an ordinary, prudent manager would exercise in the same or similar circumstances. Recently, a number of states have passed laws that allow for-profit and not-for-profit corporations to amend their articles of incorporation to limit or eliminate directors' liability for breach of the duty of care when they act in good faith.[5]

ETHICAL OBLIGATIONS OF TRUSTEES AND DIRECTORS

Legal standards represent a minimum standard of performance. What are the ethical obligations of trustees and directors? The AHA guidelines shown in Figure 6 assist in helping governing body members avoid conflicts of interest. The primary emphasis is on disclosure—putting other governing body members on notice as to a potential or actual conflict. In *Sibley,* it is uncertain that this would have made a difference, however. The "trustees" must have been aware of their colleagues' outside affiliations and activities. Adopting the AHA's statement and having knowledge of its content, however, might have alerted them to the ethical unacceptability of self-dealing and mismanagement. A conflict of interest statement would probably have made no difference as to the problem of nonmanagement because the "trustees" did not take seriously their fiduciary duty to invest hospital funds prudently.

Health services managers have characteristics of fiduciaries. They are also moral agents, and an important part of their work is to assist the organization, through the governing body, to meet its ethical and legal obligations. Concomitant with this effort, managers have a duty to help the governing body avoid conflicts of interest and problems of nonmanagement. Managers are the conscience of the organization, and they provide a stimulus to recognize ethical problems and to act in a timely fashion to avoid them or minimize their effect.

Hermann Hospital

A scandal uncovered in early 1985 involved activities of both administrators and trustees of the Hermann Hospital, an 800-bed facility, and the Hermann Hospital Estate, a trust established in 1914 to provide charity care to the poor of Houston. Investigation of the two entities showed evidence of theft, kickbacks, insider stock deals, lavish perquisites and expenditures, and expensive trips taken at the expense of the trust by trust and hospital executives and employees. Examples included allegations that the former executive director of Hermann Hospital paid money to his mistress for work never done, and that he received kickbacks from overcharges paid by Hermann Hospital to a company of which he was president. The trust filed suit against the former hospital executive director, asking that he repay $100,000 in kickbacks, $500,000 it claims he paid to his pregnant mistress, and other funds it says he laundered. The suit also alleged that he took improper trips that, along with related expenses, cost the hospital $250,000. It further alleged that he used Hermann Hospital's name, credit, and money to create an interior decorating firm for his mistress, most or all of whose income came from the hospital.

The Hermann Hospital Estate's former executive director was alleged to have stolen over $300,000. Charges against a trust employee include allegations that a luxury automobile was traded in at less than 20% of its market value for a new automobile paid for by the trust. The undervalued automobile was then purchased by the employee for the grossly understated price. In addition, there was evidence that trustees and employees had been entertained lavishly at trust expense, with records showing that $10,000 was spent by six persons on a 4-day California weekend. Newspaper accounts revealed that the Hermann Estate actually spent less than 3% of its funds on charity cases.

As a result of the investigation, two of the trustees and eight high-ranking trust and hospital executives resigned. Three persons connected with the estate, including a trustee, have been indicted on criminal charges.[6]

Many of the activities at the Hermann Hospital Estate and Hermann Hospital were unethical because they broke the law. But the misconduct goes beyond a breach of that minimum standard. The trustees violated their fiduciary duty to protect trust assets, and in this regard they squandered funds that were to have been spent to treat the poor. True trustees and directors alike are allowed no hint of conflicts of interest or of improper benefit from their association with an organization. Similarly, hospital managers must behave in a manner above reproach. They act unethically when there is self-dealing, or when assets of the organization are diverted, whether or not these are criminally indictable actions.

Cedars of Lebanon Hospital

Unlike Sibley, but like Hermann Hospital, circumstances at the Cedars of Lebanon Hospital involved a hospital administrator who engaged in both unethical and criminal behavior. The latter resulted in a prison term. As noted, criminal behavior is in itself unethical. In addition to conflict of interest, the case contains instances of self-dealing, bribery, and failure to obey federal laws. A summary of transactions in which the hospital CEO, Sanford Bronstein, engaged outlines the problems:

- Owned a consulting firm in the Caribbean with which the hospital contracted for architectural consulting services that were never performed
- Falsified board minutes to cover the fraudulent contract with his own consulting firm
- Received over 2,500 shares of stock with a market value of $75,000 in a computer company from which the hospital had purchased a $1.8 million diagnostic computer to be used for multiphasic screening. Later, underutilization of the equipment caused a loss of over $2,000 per day.

- Bribed public officials to get approval for construction and loans for an unneeded addition to the hospital
- Attempted to ease the hospital's desperate cash flow situation by not paying federal withholding on employees' salaries [7]

There are numerous other violations of ethical principles, but these are illustrative. As a result of the director's activities, the hospital was forced into receivership; the CEO was convicted and sent to prison. An important lesson in the Cedars of Lebanon case is that the governing body paid grossly insufficient attention to the CEO's activities.

CODES OF ETHICS ON CONFLICTS OF INTEREST

The American College of Healthcare Executives (ACHE) Code

The issue given most attention in the ACHE Code is conflict of interest. The section begins by stating: "A conflict of interest may be only a matter of degree . . . ."[8] This suggests that certain behavior, if limited, is unlikely to cause, or is presumed not to cause, a problem. When that same behavior becomes exaggerated, however, a conflict may arise. Gratuities provide an example in applying this criterion. There is little suggestion of a conflict of interest when a manager is treated to lunch in the cafeteria by an equipment salesman. A 2-week, all expense-paid vacation suggests something very different. Extravagant gifts or kickbacks are presumed to encourage or reward certain behavior. Nonetheless, the appearance of a conflict of interest can result by accepting *any* gratuity from those with whom business is done—even to the extent of a small gift or inexpensive lunch.

Earlier, conflict of interest was defined as the existence of duties and obligations, meeting one of which causes derogation of another. The ACHE Code defines conflict of interest more narrowly. A conflict of interest exists "when the healthcare executive: is in a position to benefit directly or indirectly by using authority or inside information, or allows a friend, relative or associate to benefit from such authority or information" or when the healthcare executive "uses authority or information to make a decision to intentionally affect the organization in an adverse manner."[9]

To minimize conflicts of interest and to eliminate them once they occur, the ACHE Code recommends mechanisms such as making all decisions in the best interests of the organization and those served by it, avoidance, and disclosure to the appropriate authority. These guidelines rely on the manager's judgment. Only the manager has the knowledge about personal activities *and* those of the organization to determine when potential or actual conflicts are present, when a solution is required, or when facts should be brought to the attention of the organization.

The American College of
Health Care Administrators (ACHCA) Code

The Code of Ethics of the American College of Health Care Administrators (ACHCA) provides some assistance for managers in solving conflicts of interest. Affiliates may not "participate in activities that reasonably may be thought to create a conflict of interest or have the potential to have a substantial adverse impact on the facility or its residents."[10] Affiliates are expected to "disclose to the governing body or other authority as may be appropriate, any actual or potential circumstance concerning him or her that might reasonably be thought to create a conflict of interest or have a substantial adverse impact on the facility or its residents."[11]

CONFLICTS OF INTEREST IN MANAGED CARE

The potential for conflicts of interest is inherent in managed care plans because the goals, purposes, and objectives of plan management and personnel may be at variance with the interests of patients (members). The tension between the plan and its members and potential members may occur as early as the marketing stage, when benefits packages and market segments are identified. Although the potential for conflicts of interests is unavoidable, their presence and consequent negative effects can be minimized, provided they are recognized and kept in mind by clinicians and managers alike.

How do conflicts of interest affect the marketing of a plan's activity? The potential conflicts of interest that exist when there is no relationship between the provider and those to whom marketing is directed can lead to actual conflicts later. This potential for conflicts is exacerbated by the fact that many plans have a self-image that is more public-service oriented and morally demanding than is typical for health services organizations. Historically, the perception of prepaid health plans and health maintenance organizations (HMOs), for example, has been that they are a "purer" delivery system—untainted by the profit motive—and one through which members gain access to high-quality medical services at moderate cost. Even though the field is changing as the number of for-profit HMOs increase, the earlier perception continues. To the extent that marketing ignores or purposely excludes high-risk groups (cream skimming), there is a variance between historic and current mission and purpose.

Adverse Selection and the Marketing of Prepaid Plans

Marketing the plan must take into account the possible need to downplay the plan's strengths. If a plan is, or is perceived to be, a leader in performing a certain technique or in treating a certain medical condition and this fact becomes known, it is likely there will be adverse selection—the plan will be inundated with new patients needing that treatment. Since higher quality may result in higher costs, the plan may also get into a vicious cycle, as a good reputation for high quality (and good results) causes more high-risk persons (who may need expensive care) to join the plan. As the plan finds itself straining against this adverse selection problem, quality may diminish for other patients, or it may have to restrict benefits or increase premiums. Thus, in order for the plan to survive, marketing may have to minimize references to outstanding care in specific areas and, instead, to focus on being seen as a place where medical services of acceptable quality are delivered, but where nothing exceptional is available.

I Want to See Dr. Nightengale

Dr. Nightengale is a pediatrician with HMO, Inc., which is located in a medium-size city. Although she had had no specialty training beyond her residency, she has proved to be a particularly adept diagnostician, often diagnosing cases that baffled her colleagues.

At the last open enrollment, plan management noted that an unusually high number of young families with children had enrolled. As is typical, there are limits on in-area, out-of-plan services and there are restrictions on referrals to subspecialists. Dr. Nightengale uses subspecialists extensively, but her results are excellent. Management's new member survey showed that for many families, the presence of excellent pediatric care was an important reason for joining HMO, Inc. Only a few named Dr. Nightengale specifically, however.

Members of management expressed fears that such perceptions might lead to an adverse selection problem among new members. It was even suggested that a special review of Dr. Nightengale's use of specialists should be undertaken in order to protect the plan's financial position. Some managers thought this was overreacting. It was agreed they would take a "wait and see" attitude. If there were problems they would have to talk to her.

This case suggests the potential for problems when prepaid plans are perceived as especially effective in treating certain types of patients.

Another example of adverse selection has occurred in treating patients with AIDS. An HMO in the Washington, D.C., area has achieved a deserved reputation for providing high-quality care to AIDS patients. This information has been disseminated within the homosexual community, and homosexuals are enrolling in that HMO in disproportionate numbers. The HMO has no data showing higher costs for people with AIDS. It is generally agreed, however, that the need for hospitalization will make caring for AIDS patients expensive, even though alternative sources of treatment are increasingly available. Sicker patients require more care, and this puts prepaid providers with disproportionate numbers of such patients at a financial, and therefore competitive, disadvantage.

Utilization of Services in Prepaid Plans

As a bureaucracy, employees, clinicians, and managers have the goal of maximizing position, power, income, and rewards with the least disruption of the organization's homeostasis. Achieving these goals, especially that of maximizing income, may result in minimizing service, whether or not that is consistent with the contract between the HMO and the payor. The bureaucratic response may even be at variance with the long-term survival of the organization: Patients seek to regain or retain their health and pay as little as possible to do so. To regain or retain their health, patients want to use the plan's services as much as necessary. If patients stay well at minimum cost and use existing services efficiently, the goals of plan and patients are congruent. The situation is rarely that simple, however.

The major source of potential conflicts of interests is in utilization of services. Patients may be divided into two groups: those who are light and moderate users and those who are heavy users of services. The plan's interests and the interests of light and moderate users are generally congruent; however, to be competitive, the plan must develop means to control heavy utilizers. Even moderate utilizers are potential financial threats to plans in competitive environments, and the plan may seek to make them light utilizers in order to trim costs. In such situations, the potential for conflicts of interest is clear.

How do potential conflicts of interests, as shown by incongruent goals of plan and patient, become true conflicts of interests? Plan marketing will describe the availability of both primary and specialty services, while downplaying limits on specialty or other expensive services. Constraints may be placed on members by limiting hours and services, thus purposely creating queues, especially for treating what are likely to be self-limiting medical conditions. The public is usually unaware that lengthy waits for appointments reduce operating costs. It is unlikely to endorse a strategy of deferring treatment, even for the more than 85% of all medical complaints that are self-limiting, regardless of the clinical and economic soundness of such a policy. Most plans have an escape valve for these pressures by providing walk-in emergency services or treating walk-in patients during office hours. A furor resulted when the CEO of a major East Coast prepaid health plan admitted publicly that there was a specific policy regarding queues and noted their value in reducing demand for certain types of services. In the long term, these policies may cause disenrollment. They are effective in the short term, however.

Physician Incentives

For the patient, the more subtle, and potentially more serious, constraints imposed by prepaid plans are directed at plan physicians. Here, there is a potential conflict of interest both between the plan and the patient, and between the physician and the patient. The Hippocratic Oath requires physicians to act in the best interests of the patient. The AMA Principles of Medical Ethics state: "A physician shall be dedicated to providing competent medical services with compassion and respect for human dignity," and "A physician shall deal honestly with patients and colleagues . . . ."[12] These ethical guidelines suggest that patients' interests must be foremost in the minds of physicians as they choose the level and content of care.

The plan, however, provides the context that facilitates or inhibits how its physicians respond. Initially, there is a self-selection bias when physicians choose where to practice. Those who cannot accept the rules imposed by a plan will seek employment elsewhere. Once a physician has joined the plan, however, management can employ a range of actions, including financial disincentives and incentives, peer pressure, nonrenewal, and dismissal to modify behavior. Plans can also limit referrals (especially outside the plan) and hospitalizations, establish quotas on the number of patients that must be seen (present in staff model HMOs), and put in place a system of peer review. Peer pressure plays an important role in most of these constraints. Constraints are positive when they encourage judicious, but appropriate use of medical resources. This may account for the fact that managed care plans usually have much lower use of ancillary services and hospital days than fee-for-service providers.

When do constraints become excessive, depriving members of needed service? When do constraints infringe on the principles of nonmaleficence and beneficence? There are no simple answers to such questions because they are a function of the plan's willingness, prompted by managers acting as moral agents, to institute safeguards that balance competitiveness and financial viability with protecting the patient.

Other Plan Constraints

Besides physician-oriented constraints, other types of constraints are found in the organizational and managerial functioning of plans. By having a complicated process (e.g., significant committee involvement and several levels of review), the plan may be slow to approve use of new procedures, techniques, or equipment that raise costs to the plan. Such complexities may be more prevalent in not-for-profit plans than in investor-owned plans. The presence of complex processes in not-for-profit plans may be a function of a greater degree of democracy, however, and not a deliberate attempt to diminish access. The effect may be the same, however. For-profit plans tend to have a narrower management pyramid and to give the CEO more authority. A complex management structure in the investor-owned plan is less likely to diminish the organization's ability to conserve resources to the potential detriment of patients.

The plan may forego purchasing high-technology equipment, or it may contract with physicians or for inpatient care of members at hospitals without such equipment. Such strategies lower costs. To the extent that lower costs enhance financial integrity and guarantee continued availability of services to patients, their interests are congruent. For those who might have benefited from access to the technology, however, there is a conflict between the interests of the patient and those of the plan.

Utilization controls such as using primary-care physicians as case managers, limiting out-of-plan services, and specifying dollar limits on referrals and consultations are useful, but plans in competitive environments must show that patients needing certain services will get them—or at least create such a perception—lest they lose market share. There is also the risk of malpractice suits and bad publicity should policies limiting utilization result in bad outcomes.

Minimizing Conflicts of Interest

How do plans and their managers prevent, or at least reduce, conflicts of interests? An indispensable first step is a willingness to acknowledge that potential conflicts of interests are inherent in the relationship between managed care plans and patients, as well as between physicians and the plan and physicians and patients. Awareness enables avoidance of many conflicts. Beyond that, checks and balances are needed. One solution is to offer the services of an ombudsman or consumer relations specialist to members. In addition, there are due process procedures for members who wish to have a matter reviewed. The success of such programs depends on enlightened management and on the personal characteristics of those involved. Plans may use the managing physician or gatekeeper concept to determine whether the patient receives needed services. Such a role may conflict with financial and other incentives constraining the plan's physicians, however. Federally qualified HMOs, for example, must have an effective grievance procedure for members. This requirement provides some protection, but for it to be useful, the member must know, or at least suspect, that care has been inadequate. This is a task the patient may be incapable of performing.

Independent audits of utilization review data developed in the plan, as well as audits of comparable data from similar plans, are means by which management determines that utilization is within acceptable limits. Internal and external comparisons such as these alert plan managers to problems in delivery of services that may result from conflicts of interests. Awareness of how conflicts of interest arise will help prevent them or minimize their effect. Such activities are essential if managers are to meet their ethical obligations to patients.

ACCEPTANCE OF GIFTS

Health services organizations must help their employees avoid conflicts of interest by adopting policies to guide their decision making. If they fail to receive guidance, employees (and managers) will perform in a fashion they believe to be reasonable. This may or may not make them more objective.

Bits and Pieces

John Henry Williams liked his new job in the radiology department of Affiliated Nursing Homes and Rehabilitation Center. He had been appointed acting head when his predecessor, Mary Beth Jacobson, went on 6 months maternity leave. John Henry would be responsible for two and a half technicians, an appointments clerk, and $250,000 in equipment. He would have authority to purchase radiographic supplies, including certain types of film. The annual value of these purchases was about $90,000. Most were obtained from three vendors, companies from which the Center had bought for years.

As Mary Beth oriented John Henry, she emphasized how much she liked the meetings with sales reps from the three vendors. Over the years, one had become a friend. Most of the meetings, she said, were held at the nice restaurant near the Center. Some were held in her office and, if so, the reps always brought along a "little something." When John Henry asked what she meant, Mary Beth gave some examples: perfume, a bottle of French brandy, and a pen set in a leather case. John Henry remembered thinking that his wife would like the perfume, but he was more interested in the lunches. It would be a chance to get away from the dreary cafeteria, as well as his boring bag lunches. Mary Beth described the lunches as nothing too fancy. She estimated the cost to the sales rep as the same as the small gifts—in the $40–$50 range.

John Henry asked Mary Beth whether there was a policy about accepting gifts from vendors. Mary Beth was put out by the question, which implied something might be wrong with what she was doing. She responded curtly that the Center trusted its managers and allowed them discretion in such matters.

John Henry asked if accepting gratuities might suggest to other staff that her decisions were influenced by the pecuniary relationship with the sales reps. Mary Beth's anger flashed. "I know you think that this thing doesn't look right. That isn't fair! I work long hours as a manager and get paid very little extra. It takes more effort and time to order and maintain proper inventory. If things go wrong, it's my head in a noose. These gifts make me feel better about my efforts. My work has been exemplary. I'd be happy to talk to anyone who thinks otherwise!!"

This case describes a problem common in many health services organizations. Several facts support Mary Beth's position. Taking clients to lunch and providing small gifts is common in business relationships. There is seemingly no cost to the organization—everything is paid by the sales representatives, who charge it to an expense account. At least one sales representative has become a friend, and Mary Beth enjoys his company socially. There is little likelihood that Mary Beth's judgment could be influenced by the small amounts of money involved. It must be asked, however, whether other vendors are being ignored because of what might be characterized as a cozy relationship.

Lacking here is any guidance from an organizational policy. Neither the ACHE nor the ACHCA Codes addresses the more subtle aspects of conflicts of interest. For example, the ACHE Code prohibits accepting "gifts or benefits offered with the expectation of influencing a management decision." Applying this provision requires that one be able to judge the giver's motivation, which is difficult, if not impossible. It is more likely that the external evidence, including the benefits offered and accepted, will have to be the basis for the conclusion about a conflict.

A decision maker gains or has the potential to gain from conflicts of interest in many ways. Often ignored are circumstances in which the parties understand that in the future the decision maker will be considered favorably for employment or other benefits. A promise or suggestion of future gain creates potential or actual conflicts of interest, and should be included in prohibitions cited in the code. Classic nonhealth sector examples of these circumstances are common. Military personnel on active duty interact with contractors and suppliers; on retirement, they accept employment with the same organizations. Similarly, former members of Congress and staff of federal agencies find lucrative employment as lobbyists or as employees of organizations they formerly affected. The occurrence of such problems in the health services field is more than a hypothetical possibility, and its likelihood increases as health care becomes increasingly politicized and as large aggregations of health services organizations become common.

Anyone who takes something of value knowing the giver intends to influence the recipient acts unethically. Bribery is a clear-cut example—the recipient knows what is being done and what is being bought. The typical relationship of giver and recipient is more subtle, however. What does the pharmacy director do about the proffered lunch from the drug detailer? Does the CEO stop a dietitian from accepting a basket of holiday fruits and nuts from the greengrocer? What about the modest gift from the equipment salesman who was the successful bidder during the renovation program completed 3 years earlier? Or 10 years earlier? Such transactions suggest potential conflicts of interest. The gift might be given with the intent of receiving special consideration in the future, or might be payment for past decision making.

Such situations become even more complex because it is difficult to distinguish the activities of managers and staffs from normal interactions. People develop relationships and friendships, whether as buyer and seller or as professional colleagues. If such is the case, however, one should expect the buyer to be equally generous in providing gifts to the seller.

All health services organizations should prospectively address the question of gratuities. Such a policy can follow one of three options. One is an absolute prohibition on accepting gifts, regardless of value. This is the policy endorsed by the American Society for Hospital Materials Management in its Code of Ethics, which states: "Decline all gifts or gratuities and do not enter into any transactions that would result in . . . personal benefit."[13] This policy may cause stress for employees who feel awkward declining gifts of trivial value. However, the policy is straightforward and simple; no judgment is required. This clear, unequivocal rule justifies refusing all gifts and this adds much to its usefulness.

The second option is pragmatic, but because judgment and occasional difficult decisions are involved, applying it is more complex. A criterion of reasonableness is applied to the examples given above. This criterion allows for a variety of circumstances, and recognizes that persons in organizations have friends and relationships. What must be assiduously avoided is any hint of wrongdoing or conflict of interest in decision making, however. As previously noted, this is difficult to achieve. The test should be what the reasonable person objectively viewing the situation would conclude about the intent of the giver and the effect of a gift on the manager.

A third option—a hybrid of the first two—is a compromise for organizations that prefer not to enforce an absolute prohibition, but want to minimize conflict of interest and aid employees who need the support of a rule. Under this policy, all gifts, however insignificant, are considered as gifts to the organization. They are made available for its use by turning them into the materials manager, either for redistribution to staff or for other corporate uses. If given to the organization, or widely shared with staff, the potential for personal conflict of interest ceases to exist, even though there may continue to be conflict between the organization and patients.

Option three is similar to a health services organization that receives gifts from investor-owned businesses. It is common for suppliers of goods and services to make cash or in-kind contributions to not-for-profit organizations. Accepting such gifts is not considered a conflict of interest. The contribution benefits the organization directly and as a whole, just as a price cut or a discount would. It does not benefit one individual, even though the reflected glory of such contributions may enhance the reputations of those managing the organization at that time.

Only a Matter of Degree

Stimson received four Super Bowl tickets in the mail. Attached was a note from the local sales representative for a major equipment manufacturing company. It read: "Thought you might be able to use these." The nursing facility (NF) of which Stimson is CEO recently decided it should build a major addition to house a rehabilitation unit. The representative's company manufactures equipment that could be used in the facility. Stimson had called the manufacturer several months earlier to discuss equipment that might be available in order to make the specifications for the bidding process more precise.

Stimson is in a difficult situation. Super Bowl tickets are expensive and difficult to obtain, but their value is subjective. Although Super Bowl tickets are generally highly prized, some recipients would place little value on them. Absent a personal relationship, such as a long-standing friendship, the tickets seem to be intended to affect the CEO's decision. Important in discussing this is whether Stimson is the sole proprietor and the NF is operated for profit. If so, Stimson's interests and those of the organization are one—there can be no economic conflict of interest. Nonetheless, the owner's financial interests may conflict with interests of the NF's residents. This is a different type of conflict of interest.

APPROVAL OF SELF-DIRECTED EXPENDITURE

More subtle questions of conflict of interest can be self-induced. It seems a safe assumption that the health services manager typically identifies a personal obligation to put patient interests before their own. How much, then, should be spent to refurbish the CEO's office suite? What type of automobile should the organization lease for the CEO? Answers to these questions vary by type of organization and its ownership.

Patient or Self?

Anderson is the CEO of Community Hospital, a private, not-for-profit organization. It is well managed by Anderson and an effective administrative staff. Because the results of Anderson's management have been good year after year, the governing body interferes little in the internal operations, and spends almost all of its time on fundraising and community relations. Anderson has a large discretionary fund, which can be used for any purpose. In the past, it has been used for entertainment, gifts, and staff educational activities.

At the urging of several governing body members and managers, Anderson redecorated the administrative suite. Rosewood and leather sofas were ordered, a burled oak desk installed, and several original oil paintings selected by the interior decorator. Cost estimates of the project exceeded $50,000.

When criticism of these costs began to surface even among the more financially successful members of the medical staff,

Anderson reacted defensively. The primary argument made by Anderson to justify the expenditure was that the CEO of a multi-million dollar enterprise must have the accoutrements of office to be effective. Few of the critics was placated.

The appropriateness of an expenditure such as this will vary by context and setting. A heavily endowed private hospital, in which the CEO's office is expected to reflect success and sophistication, will view this case differently from a charity hospital in which each nickel is spent reluctantly. For organizations at either extreme, however, it is easy to note that $50,000 could fund worthwhile projects, both administrative and clinical. No one expects the CEO to sit on orange crates and use brick and board bookshelves, but good judgment tempered by reasonableness should be the criterion. Again, a useful criterion is to try to view such actions as would an informed, objective outsider.

Conflict of Interest Without Direct Personal Gain

The case of Miriam Hospital is similar to that of Hermann Hospital. Both fall between the Sibley and Cedars of Lebanon cases. It has an element of conflict of interest; other characteristics make it unique.

Miriam Hospital

Before 1980, routine blood tests at Miriam Hospital were performed by a six-channel analyzer. In 1980, the hospital purchased and put into operation a 12-channel analyzer. Because of a computer programming error, patients continued to be charged for both sets of tests, even though only the 12-channel machine was used.

A year later, Blue Cross raised questions about the unusually high laboratory charges at Miriam compared with other hospitals. The explanation was that doctors at Miriam simply ordered more lab tests. In 1982, a Professional Standards Review Organization (PSRO) audit clerk uncovered the double billing. The manager of information systems was ordered by his immediate superior to eliminate the programming error. Shortly thereafter, however, he was told by top officials at Miriam to reinstate the programming error.

Later in 1982, a Blue Cross auditor uncovered the same problem and asked for a copy of the program. The manager of data processing was told to erase any evidence in the program that showed that the original error had been reintroduced. Blue Cross was given the sanitized program.

Shortly thereafter, two data-processing personnel were accused of allowing an outside company to use Miriam's computer in contravention of hospital policy. Each was offered the opportunity to resign. Fearing he would be made a scapegoat, one of them went to Blue Cross with the information. Blue Cross took the case to the attorney general's office. Six months later, a grand jury handed down indictments of the hospital and several senior managers. The charges included: obtaining money under false pretenses, conspiracy, and filing false documents. The alleged overbilling totalled almost $2.8 million.

The hospital's and managers' defense was based on their interpretation of the rules under which reimbursement was made. They argued that the rules required hospitals to continue with the same accounting methods for the entire fiscal year, even though there were errors of the sort found in this case. An end-of-fiscal-year audit would determine what financial adjustments were needed.[14]

Unlike the Cedars of Lebanon and Hermann Hospital cases, there is no evidence here that managers gained personally from their action. Miriam Hospital was the only direct beneficiary of the double billing. This does not excuse the action, ethically or legally, but does put it in a different light. Unlike the Sibley Hospital case, these executives did not benefit other organizations to the hospital's detriment. Nonetheless, to the extent that they improved the hospital's financial situation, the managers enhanced their own positions at Miriam. They thus benefited through continued employment, enhanced status and reputation, and, perhaps, financial rewards from the organization. Miriam Hospital's financial position is unclear; some sources stated that it could not afford to refund the overcharges, although management reported that this was not a problem. Saving a financially troubled organization at personal risk is altruistic and self-sacrificing; such efforts, however, also benefit the managers. Nonetheless, selfless or self-sacrificing activities cannot overshadow moral values and ethical codes. The end cannot be used to justify the means.

SYSTEMS CONFLICTS

Typically, health services managers serve on boards of health-related organizations. Examples include health planning agencies, charities, insurance companies, Blue Cross plans, HMOs, and hospital associations. Inherent in such service is a distinct potential for conflicts of interests. Neither the ACHE nor the ACHCA code provides any guidance in this regard. If a conflict does exist, participation must cease. This action is similar to that suggested by the AHA and ACHE for conflicts of interest. However, dramatic changes in the health services environment may have made these precautions inadequate.

The present dilemma originated with the manager's civic duty and professional responsibilities to assist communities in meeting their health needs. These efforts are reinforced by the provisions of various codes of ethics, as well as the orientation of governing bodies. Although health services managers should be encouraged to apply their professional expertise to improving the efficiency and effectiveness of community health services, the potential for conflicts of interest is apparent. It can be present even though other health services providers are not being discussed. If the health services manager is also a Blue Cross director, for example, there is a potential conflict over rates, programs, and covered services. Furthermore, in some areas, Blue Cross is becoming a competitor and developing health services delivery programs. Although the manager abstains from voting on decisions directly affecting the manager's organization, there is no way to avoid becoming privy to corporate thinking and strategies of other activities that in general, as well as specific, ways may affect that manager's health services organization. Once known, this knowledge cannot be ignored by the manager.

With increasing competitiveness in the health services field, all information about one's competitors is important to meet perceived or actual threats to market share or to blunt an unfriendly initiative. In fact, duties of fidelity and loyalty to the organization require managers to act effectively to preserve or expand market share. If managers minimize the problem of conflict through disclosure and withdrawal when necessary, they will diminish their effectiveness. Furthermore, they open themselves to charges of acting improperly because of the likely appearance of impropriety.

How is this problem solved? How does the health services organization obtain important expertise without exposing itself and manager-members to charges of impropriety? One answer is to permit service only by persons from noncompeting organizations. This solution has the disadvantage of potentially excluding persons with operational experience in that geographic area. However, over time out-of-area directors will develop needed expertise. This solution is complicated by the growing number of vertically or horizontally integrated multi-institutional organizations, which replace the traditional, locally-based organization with one with statewide or national activities.

There are two other solutions. Health services organizations may use full-time directors—persons who serve as directors only of noncompeting organizations and who have no other employment. Full-time directors are common in business enterprise, but rare in health services, especially in the not-for-profit sector. These individuals are usually paid—an expenditure that should pose no problem for health services organizations, especially the larger ones. Those unable to bear the cost should consider option three.

The third option uses services of professionally prepared and experienced persons not actively managing health services organizations. Examples include retired health services managers and health services administration educators. Physicians and well-informed members of the public could serve effectively. This option has most of the advantages of option two with few disadvantages. Here, too, an economic relationship is desirable, since it is likely to produce more commitment and higher quality involvement.

Managers working to improve community health services through cooperative efforts face an environment that is increasingly competitive. This makes some types of cooperation difficult or impossible. Other types of cooperation, such as sharing services and participating in joint ventures, are stimulated. Survival is a major corporate goal for all health services organizations, and new ethical guidelines are needed to help address these problems.

CONCLUSION

Avoiding conflicts of interest requires constant vigilance. Managers of government-owned facilities risk fines and criminal charges if they are involved in conflicts of interest. The likelihood of legal penalties is smaller in the private sector. This does not obviate the ethical problem, however. Disclosure to eliminate or minimize the problem is stressed by the ACHE, ACHCA, and AHA. This presumes that one recognizes potential conflicts. Failure to recognize such conflicts means that managers are well into a conflict situation before they realize it. Conflicts of interest can be very subtle, and continual questioning and self-analysis are needed to identify them. Their potential and actual effect will increase as competition intensifies.

In addition to disclosure, there are several other ways to avoid or eliminate conflicts of interest. They include divestiture of an outside interest that might cause a conflict, seeking guidance from the governing body when questions arise, and not participating in or attempting to influence any matter in which a conflict of interest might exist. Such steps eliminate the conflict or put the governing body on notice. Both are important. But it is managers who must realize that moral agency is inherent in the profession, and they must continually work to minimize the risk of conflict of interest or eliminate it once it is present.

Systems conflicts will cause unique problems as well as open up opportunities in the new competitive environment. To avoid conflicts of interest, managers will have to be especially alert, and may have to withdraw from all involvement in governing and advising health services organizations. Nontraditional means will be required to maximize the assistance that persons experienced in health services can offer, while at the same time minimizing the potential for systems conflicts.

NOTES

1. Harlan Cleveland, *The Future Executive* (New York: Harper & Row, 1972), 104.

2. Arthur F. Southwick, *The Law of Hospital and Health Care Administration,* 2nd ed. (Ann Arbor, Michigan: Health Administration Press, 1988), 123–126.

3. 381 Federal Supplement 1003 (1974).

4. Ibid., 1013.

5. Thomas M. Collins, "Trustees and Personal Liability: The Good News," *Trustee 41* (September 1988): 18–19.

6. *Houston Post,* articles dated March 5, 9, 10, 12, 13, 16, and 19, 1985, and *Washington Post,* March 21, 1985.

7. Summarized from a case study written by Milton C. Devolites, Professor Emeritus, Department of Health Services Administration, The George Washington University, Washington, D.C. The case was prepared from various issues of the *Miami Herald* and *Miami News* in 1974.

8. American College of Healthcare Executives, "Code of Ethics," 1988.

9. Ibid.

10. American College of Health Care Administrators, "Code of Ethics," 1989.

11. Ibid.

12. American Medical Association, "Principles of Medical Ethics," 1980.

13. American Society for Hospital Materials Management, "Code of Ethics," October 19, 1980.

14. *Providence Journal-Bulletin,* articles dated September 22, 1983; October 2, 5, and 6, 1983; and May 16, 1984.

7

∞

ETHICAL DUTIES TOWARD
THE ORGANIZATION

THIS CHAPTER IDENTIFIES SEVERAL administrative ethical issues arising from the manager's interactions with the organization. Most prominent are handling of confidential and insider information, self-dealing, and the appropriate relationship between the manager and the governing body and medical staff. In the course of their duties, health services managers are privy to a great deal of confidential information, some of which is of a proprietary nature. This type of information is to be distinguished from that collected, used, and maintained for purposes of patient care. The proper handling of confidential information should be of major concern to the health services organization. This issue has received relatively little attention, however.

A major part of this chapter is devoted to the manager's role in resource allocation, which has ethical implications for both the organization and the community. The era of limited resources means that health services organizations and their managers must prospectively determine how resources are allocated. The background provided here should assist them to do so.

PROPER HANDLING OF CONFIDENTIAL INFORMATION

Patient Records

The manager's first ethical obligation is to protect the patient's medical record. Ethical and legal requirements are clear here. Organizations have a legal duty to keep medical records confidential and secure. Critical for good patient care, these records must be legible, current, complete, and authenticated. This is done by providing adequate and effective personnel, systems, and procedures in medical records activities, and by ensuring that medical staff bylaws and rules and regulations are enforced. In terms of medical record security, much can be done to prevent or minimize unauthorized access. Whatever are the legal requirements that pertain—and these vary from state to state—managers have an ethical duty to ensure the confidentiality of all patients' medical records.

The most common breach of this ethic results from discussing patients' medical conditions with persons who have no need to know. Idle talk and gossip about patients may be titillating, but is absolutely inappropriate both inside and outside the health services organization.

In some instances, maintaining confidential information about patients and furthering organizational interests conflict.

Mailing Lists

University Hospital has a very active cardiac medicine section in its department of medicine. Over several decades it has treated thousands of persons with heart problems ranging from angina to congestive heart failure. Its patients have been included in several study protocols, many of which have been funded by the National Institutes of Health (NIH) or a national heart association.

As part of long-term patient follow-up, regular questionnaire surveys are conducted. In order to perform these surveys, extensive mailing lists are maintained by the cardiac medicine section. On one occasion the development office of University Hospital used the mailing list to solicit general contributions. On another occasion, it undertook a special fundraising effort to assist in converting and equipping a six-bed cardiac intensive care unit. Contributions by the cardiac program's present and former patients have been excellent, primarily because of the program's superior rapport with and reputation among patients.

The physician director of the program and her administrative assistant have been approached by a prominent national life insurance company, which has been impressed with the results of the program. It wants to market life insurance to the program's participants. The proposal is attractive because the opportunity to obtain life insurance will benefit present and former patients, since many of them are otherwise uninsurable except at very high premiums, and because any data obtained by the insurance company will be available to the hospital at cost if the mailing list is provided to the insurance company.

The physician director and administrative assistant are very enthusiastic about the clinical possibilities (in addition to the opportunity of helping patients). The director of development sees the sale of mailing lists as a means of raising money for the cardiac program's activities. Both he and the physician director have just spent an hour trying to convince the CEO about the appropriateness of releasing the mailing list for this worthy purpose.

This case suggests the legitimate but opposing and competing considerations involved in patient care, research, fundraising, and a general duty of beneficence to help patients solve problems not directly linked to medical treatment.

The case is used here to highlight ethical problems surrounding patient information. Using the information in the way suggested violates the confidentiality of patient treatment and diagnosis. There may be some direct benefit to patients (because of the opportunity provided to obtain life insurance) and some indirect benefits to the organization (through improved data for epidemiological studies). Nonetheless, using the mailing lists serves no true research purpose, nor does it directly further the patients' medical treatment. Data that do not specifically identify patients serve the same epidemiological purposes. The promise of mortality data on insurance purchasers is incidental to the research effort, and the money earned selling the mailing list is likely to be modest. In any event, these utilitarian arguments are not relevant, because such uses are incompatible with the principle of respect for persons, which includes the right to privacy. Using the list to solicit contributions was inappropriate, and should thus not be used as an argument for making the list available in other ways.

A weightier argument for using mailing lists could be made if all University Hospital patients were included, rather than singling out patients with a particular diagnosis. Mailing to all former patients identifies only that the person has been a patient at the hospital. Even this may be violating some patients' privacy, however. This problem may be minimized by asking patients on admission whether they object to having their names on mailing lists used for hospital purposes, such as fundraising.

Hospital use of lists must be distinguished from sale or rental of the mailing lists. If it is the hospital's intent to use the list commercially, patients must be so informed. (Obtaining consent raises numerous questions, which are discussed in Chapter 9.) Patients' privacy concerns may change over time, and patients should be informed of their right to have their names removed from such lists at any time. Rental or sale of mailing lists in the medical setting is fraught with ethical difficulties and is probably best avoided. Even if lists are used internally, care must be taken to avoid any breach of confidentiality.

Organizational Information

In addition to patient information, the manager is privy to confidential information (also known as proprietary information) about the organization. As with patient information, a basic criterion for use of confidential information is the need to know. Examples of confidential information include the organization's development plans, its plans for new equipment purchases, its business and marketing strategies, its plans for medical staff development, and its financial and personnel programs. Equally important, but less commonly included, are general information about the staff and organization, and specific information about particular managers or governing body members. Making any confidential information available to unauthorized organizations or persons—either deliberately or through negligence—is unethical.

In a competitive environment, loose lips can cause significant adverse consequences. It is unethical to provide confidential information to unauthorized persons or organizations, whether or not the manager's organization is put directly at risk or experiences a loss, and whether or not the manager making the communication gains personally.

The American College of Healthcare Executives (ACHE) Code directs the healthcare executive to "respect professional confidences." This wording is regrettably vague, and provides insufficient guidance about confidential organizational information. Managers as well as members of the governing body and the medical staff throughout the organization must ensure that confidential information is safeguarded. Medical staff members are especially difficult to control, and acute care hospitals are increasingly providing information to them on a need-to-know basis.

MISUSE OF INSIDER INFORMATION AND SELF-DEALING

Ethical problems concerning the organization's confidential information arise when managers use it in a manner that is inconsistent with their fiduciary duty (duty of trust) to the organization. Persons in the organization who have access to information not available to the public are known as insiders.

Problems with insider (confidential) information arise when such information is used for self-dealing, or for the benefit of associates of the manager. Confidential information is also misused, for example, when all internal efforts have failed, and the manager has no choice morally but to make public information about unsafe practices that affect patient safety. Here, however, the manager's duty of moral agency to protect the patient takes precedence and must be met—even though doing so violates a lesser moral obligation and may subject the manager to civil or criminal sanctions.

Narrowly defined, self-dealing occurs only when a person with access to confidential information uses it for purposes of self-aggrandizement, such as monetary gain or other advantage. Misuse of confidential information that does not involve self-dealing is considered simply a breach of confidentiality. Examples of misuse of insider information include: a manager, knowing that the organization intends to establish a surgicenter in a specific location, purchases the property through a dummy corporation or a straw man, and later resells it to the organization for a profit; a manager discloses information about organization decision making that helps his associates do business with the organization; and a manager discloses market strategies (proprietary information) to competitors, with no resulting personal gain. If, in the first example, the manager is decision maker for both the sale and the purchase, a conflict of interest is present as well.

What's a Manager to Do?

S.L. Rine joined the managerial staff of a large health services provider after working elsewhere for several years. Rine is an affiliate of the American College of Healthcare Executives (ACHE), and wants to build the best set of credentials in the shortest possible time. Rine wants to become a CEO.

Rine is responsible for several support departments, as well as some clinical areas. Shortly after joining the organization, he realized that it was very political. Much of what happens at the senior level is the result of personal relationships and obligations.

One of Rine's departments—maintenance—is responsible for all grounds. Rine found that grounds crews were being sent to homes of senior members of the board to maintain their lawns, shrubs, and trees. Rine asked the maintenance director to explain, and was told that the practice had a long history and that things were better left as they were. When Rine asked the director for a cost estimate of the grounds work being done at the private homes, the director refused to provide it, and said he wasn't about to incur the wrath of the board members who were benefiting. Rine pondered what to do.

Shortly after talking to the maintenance director, Rine had lunch with the laboratory director. Without discussing the specifics, Rine described the problem in maintenance. The laboratory director exclaimed, "That's nothing!", and went on to describe how two board members were selling reagents, supplies, and equipment to the laboratory at what she believed were higher than market prices. Rine asked the laboratory director if she had done anything about the situation. She replied that her predecessor has tried to stop the practice and was fired for his trouble. Rine pondered what to do.

This case has two dimensions—one involving governing body members, the other involving managers. Board members whose yards are maintained by the organization or who sell supplies to the laboratory at inflated prices are using their special relationship with the organization for personal gain. Explicitly or implicitly, they are using their authority in an improper manner. Selling overpriced supplies to the laboratory seems more unethical than providing free yard maintenance to board members. Both, however, improperly divert (steal) organizational resources. In principle, there is no difference between the two acts. Most destructive for the moral health of the organization is that the governing body members are setting a bad example, one that at the very least will make the staff cynical and at worst will encourage them to use their authority to act improperly.

The second dimension is the role of managers. Knowing about improper behavior but failing to act is little better than committing an improper act. The codes of administrative ethics are of limited help. Rine and the laboratory manager agree that the behavior is unacceptable. The dilemma they face is to identify and act on their duties. By confronting the erring managers, Rine is likely to achieve little other than embarrassing those involved. Nonetheless, there are steps managers can take. One is to question the appropriateness of unethical activities at every opportunity. Managers can encourage their colleagues to speak out. Once several managers become involved, they can draw strength from one another. They can seek to implement a policy of competitive bidding for laboratory purchases. They can seek to develop and adopt an organization-wide policy on self-dealing and abuse of power. In short, they must take whatever steps they can to end these unethical practices. As moral agents, they cannot close their eyes to the problem.

A common misuse of confidential (nonpublic) information in the business world is employees (insiders) using such information for advantageous stock market transactions. Historically, health services organizations have been largely unaffected by this problem because few were publicly traded corporations. This has changed dramatically since 1980. Regulation by the Securities and Exchange Commission or its state counterparts does not diminish the seriousness of the unethical conduct inherent in misusing insider information. Again, the law is a minimum requirement that does not necessarily set an appropriate level of ethical behavior. The following case illustrates several of these ethical problems.

Just Part Owner

John Abernathy is the CEO of a large not-for-profit NF in an urban area. For several months, the governing body's capital expenditure subcommittee has been considering the purchase of equipment to increase its capacity in rehabilitation medicine. A major recommendation of the long-range planning committee at a retreat last year had been to consider rehabilitation as a major new initiative. The facility currently has a part-time physician director of the program, but he has expressed interest in becoming full time.

Following the death of an uncle 2 years ago, Abernathy inherited 1,000 shares of INCO, Inc. stock. Abernathy voluntarily submits an annual statement of investments and holdings as part of the board's conflict of interest disclosure requirement. The next report is not due for 9 months, however. In INCO's last annual report to stockholders, Abernathy noted that 10 million shares of common stock are publicly held. One of INCO's activities is manufacturing rehabilitation equipment such as the equipment Abernathy's facility is considering purchasing.

The capital expenditure subcommittee prepared a preliminary report and gave a copy to Abernathy for review. Abernathy dislikes making private financial information available to the governing body, and is distressed about what he recognizes as the need for special disclosure.

Theoretically, Abernathy faces a conflict of interest. There is also the potential for misuse of confidential information for the purpose of self-dealing. As the decision maker, Abernathy is in a position to purchase equipment from a manufacturer in which he owns stock. Abernathy's interest is very remote—he owns a mere .01% of the company's stock—and the potential for personal gain is so small that it is not reasonable to believe that Abernathy would be influenced by his stock holdings. The objectivity of the decision becomes more suspect as the degree of interest increases. Nevertheless, Abernathy should disclose his holdings in INCO, even though it is personally repugnant.

RELATIONS WITH THE GOVERNING BODY

The CEO is hired by the governing body to act as its agent in achieving the organization's mission. In turn, the CEO selects, hires, evaluates, and retains subordinate managers. The CEO, the organization's managers, and the medical staff are all moral agents, not just morally neutral arms and legs of the organization.

It was noted earlier that some sectarian health services organizations require all managers midlevel and above to belong to the religious faith of the sponsoring organization. This requirement seems overly restrictive—even coreligionists hold different views of the rigor of application or importance of various doctrines. What is needed for an effective corporate culture is that managers (among others) have a complete understanding of the organization's philosophy, and that they accept it. It is possible to draw on humanism or a nonreligion-based philosophy to reach the same human values as those of a particular religious dogma. Culling for like values occurs in the recruiting and selection process. Ethical compatibility should be determined then also. A major advantage of this more flexible approach is that it broadens the field from which competent managers can be recruited.

The governing body and the CEO and senior management (shown in Figure 7 as "Administration") must clearly define the scope of their respective functions. Figure 7 also suggests the need to distinguish senior management from middle management. Lacking a clear understanding of their respective activities, governance, administration, and management will interfere in each other's spheres, with resulting inefficiency and frustration of organizational goals. The diagram should not be interpreted to mean that these relationships and spheres must remain discrete. There is permeability of thoughts, ideas, and communications, but, their separateness, as well as jointness, must be clear.

Historically, important writers in hospital administration argued that having the CEO or members of the medical staff on the governing body caused a great potential for conflicts of interest, and that any advantages were far outweighed by risks.[1] Current thinking, however, is that the protections offered by disclosure and sensitivity to the problem of conflicts of interest generally pre-

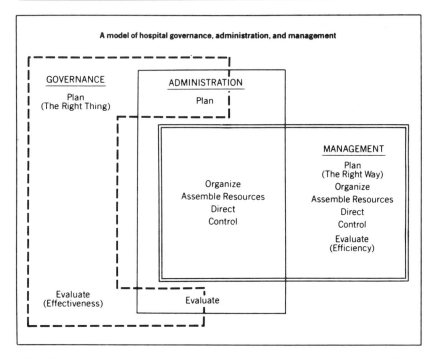

Figure 7. A model of hospital governance, administration, and management. (Reprinted from *Trustee, 34,* 6, by permission, June 1981. Copyright 1981, American Hospital Publishing, Inc.)

vent, or at least minimize, the probability of such abuses. The environment in health services has changed, and involvement in and awareness of governing body activities by the CEO and medical staff are now generally considered very important. According to an ACHE study published in 1984, "in the not-for-profit freestanding group [of hospitals], only 40 per cent of CEOs are voting members on boards. In contrast, almost two-thirds (64 per cent) of CEOs in not-for-profit (hospital) systems vote on boards. About half of all investor-owned CEOs have voting privileges."[2]

Anecdotal evidence suggests that there is a trend toward increasing the number of internal governing body members—senior managers from within the organization—relative to external members. Internal board members are considered desirable because of the expertise they bring. There is, however, undoubtedly an increased potential for conflicts of interest.

The CEO and other senior managers link the governing body and the organization as a whole, whether or not they are governing body members. Senior managers are thus able to sanitize data, develop and present it in the best light (even to the point of misleading the board, as happened at Cedars of Lebanon), and engage in similar practices to make management look good. A key issue is how much information and what types of information the governing body should receive. This must be determined by the governing body itself. As agents of the governing body, the CEO and senior managers provide the information. They may be asked for recommendations, but the governing body must be sufficiently informed to know which data it must have and how to interpret them.

Of course, managers want to cast organizational performance in the best light. Environmental changes have increased the pressure to perform. These increased pressures may tempt managers to engage in "creative reporting" about their performance.

Ethically, managers have a responsibility to be truthful in reporting to their governing bodies. This stems from the principle of respect for persons, which applies to all persons with whom the manager deals. Deception is disrespectful. This does not mean that the staff must emphasize unfavorable information—a balanced picture is prudent and desirable. It does mean that problems be presented honestly and forthrightly, and that the governing body be informed in a timely fashion. All managers must be alert to efforts to understate or misrepresent problems. The issue of truthfulness is closely related to the issue of whistleblowing, which is discussed later in this chapter. Standardizing and routinizing reporting minimizes the potential to manipulate the system or data for selfish reasons.

Appraising Managerial Performance

A major role of the governing body is to appraise the CEO's performance. The CEO appraises performance of subordinate managers. Harvey has developed an appraisal process that uses a management by objectives (MBO) format.[3] He details various competencies necessary to managerial effectiveness: planning and organizing, achieving hospital objectives, maintaining the quality of medical services, allocating resources fairly and efficiently, resolving crises, complying with regulations, and promoting the hospital. Harvey's criteria focus on hospital management performance, but could be used with any health services organization in which actual performance is compared against predetermined measures and standards. A recent survey found that 76% of governing bodies in responding hospitals formally evaluate the CEO.[4] Anecdotal evidence suggests that few CEOs are evaluated with the formality Harvey recommends, however.

To avoid conflicts of interest during the evaluation process, CEOs must limit their role to explaining organizational performance. The CEO's performance should be reviewed without the CEO present. Problems are minimized if the governing body has a formally established process for evaluating performance of the CEO—one based on predetermined objectives that are to be attained during the period under evaluation.

The following case illustrates the problem of information flow to the governing body.

I Wonder If They Even Care!

Stu White had just returned to his office from a monthly board meeting. His assistant, Barbara Jones, saw he was very agitated. Jones asked, "How did it go?" White responded by re-telling an often-repeated story about his board and the unique problems he seemed to have with it. "I believe I could tell them the moon was made of green cheese and they would believe it! They don't seem to know, or care, what happens in this nursing home." White went on to describe how he did all of the thinking for the board. When he came to the facility, there was no board reporting system. White had established one based on his pre-vious experience. He emphasized that the organization had been lucky to have honest managers, because anybody else "could have been hauling it out of here by the carload."

Here, the information flow problem results from the governing body's lack of awareness or its unwillingness to accept responsibility and accountability for the organization—a duty that is unquestionably theirs. White is in a powerful position because he can determine what information the board receives. Few managers find themselves in such a situation. However, most managers are so much better informed than their governing bodies that they necessarily serve as information conduits. This puts them in a critical position—one that can cause ethical problems. A first step for White is to educate the governing body about its responsibilities. He must then help the board to identify the data and reports it needs to meet those responsibilities.

RELATIONS WITH THE MEDICAL STAFF

The medical staff's relations with the organization and its managers have nu-merous ethical dimensions. These are present whether the organization has a matrix design or the traditional hierarchy of relationships for administrative and clinical departments. Schulz and Johnson suggest that the CEO's role has evolved from that of business manager to coordinator to corporate chief, and is now that of management team leader.[5] As a management team leader, the CEO functions as a partner with the medical staff. This is a collegial relationship, one in which peers address and solve problems of mutual concern. Regardless of the role and degree of acceptance by the medical staff, the CEO has duties and responsibilities that inevitably cause occasional disagreements with the medical staff.

Managers' most important relationships are their relationships with pa-tients, whose interests managers must protect. A conflict of duties—perhaps even a conflict of interests—arises from managers' need to maintain harmo-nious relationships with the medical staff and at the same time ensure that the patients' interests are guaranteed. Physicians, too, must meet duties of respect for persons, beneficence, and nonmaleficence. At times these principles are not met. The manager must be attentive to the needs and activities of the medical staff because physician involvement is essential to providing patient care. The physician–patient relationship is vital to the organization. But conflicts may result from enforcement of medical staff bylaws, from review of the consent process, and in the working relationships between physicians and other staff.

For several decades, it has been insufficient for managers to be concerned only with the financial aspects of the health services organization. The green eyeshade mentality is no more than an historical curiosity. Managers are now ethically (and legally) expected to be aware of clinical practice and to intervene as necessary. This broader role has positive and negative aspects. Although managers are not competent to judge the quality of clinical practice, they act through experts who are. This situation is analogous to that of a manager responsible for pharmacy or dietetics. Here, too, the manager must rely on technical expertise to assess performance and make decisions. Some physicians react negatively to even a hint of such involvement, which they see as interference in the practice of medicine. In fact, managerial involvement serves the physician's best interests as well, in that it ensures the highest quality medicine possible. Anecdotal evidence suggests that more competent physicians are least likely to object to review of their cases. What must be stressed is that the manager is not judging quality of care directly, but only in cooperation with those who are clinically competent to do so.

The late 1970s and 1980s witnessed significant changes in perceptions about relationships between physicians and health services organizations, especially acute care hospitals. A term used early in that development was *MeSH* (medical staff-hospital) organizations. The term did not gain wide acceptance, and the term *joint venture* replaced it. Joint ventures between health services organizations and physicians are designed to add an economic dimension to relationships that emphasize clinical activities. It is believed that tying physicians to the organization economically enhances the organization's ability to survive, and improves medical staff morale and commitment. Typical examples of joint ventures include professional office buildings and the lease or purchase and operation of high-technology equipment. Special attention must be paid to the ethical implications of such arrangements, however. A mildly adversarial relationship between medical staff and managers is useful because it provides checks and balances in maintaining high-quality patient care. But this requires that each party remember that its reason for being is to serve and protect the patient. When management and the medical staff are economically bound, the patient's interests may suffer. The potential for conflicts of interest is greatly increased if the physicians involved in joint ventures are also part of the governing body.

DEALING WITH FRAUDULENT CREDENTIALS

There are regular, but infrequent, reports of persons claiming to be physicians, but whose credentials have been wholly or partly falsified. The problem of overstated, misrepresented, or false credentials is extensive in the business world, and there is no reason to believe that health services management has been immune. Examples of misrepresenting credentials include: inflating job titles, responsibilities, and duties; exaggerating or falsifying academic preparation and credentials; and relating false or misleading information regarding professional achievement or activities. Such actions are dishonest and unethical.

Nonexistent credentials are relatively easy to uncover. The more subtle and more pervasive problem is "creative" resume writing. One need only look at resumes produced by some employment and executive search firms to realize that it is possible to make trivial management positions appear significant. Uncovering exaggerated or overstated credentials can be difficult because the specific details of employment must be verified. Even job descriptions may not adequately reflect what the incumbent really did in a particular position. For this reason, gray cases may slip through. Egregious examples can be identified, however.

If a manager encounters an applicant who has been dishonest in presenting credentials, the course of action is clear—exposure and disciplinary action through the professional society. The actions to be taken if one discovers that a current employee has used false or dishonestly presented credentials is less clear-cut. Having discovered such fraudulence, the manager must act to end it. Counseling the employee is a first step, whether or not the employee is to be retained. Beyond that, the action should be proportionate to the seriousness of the falsification. Current job performance and the reasons the employee falsified the credentials should also be taken into account.

What action should be taken if a manager has overstated, misrepresented, or falsified qualifications? Managers who have falsified credentials should inform their superiors about the problem and offer the strongest possible rationale for the action. This is a sound course of action even when the claimed credential does not exist, but was material to the hiring decision. The employer may not take drastic action, especially if the reasons for what was done seem compelling. Current job performance will also be considered. The manager must be prepared for termination, however. Continued concealment is unacceptable: as one becomes increasingly senior in an organization, the stakes are higher, and potential damage to one's career is greater. Misrepresented or false credentials are a burden to the individual, because they are likely eventually to be uncovered, and because there is the chronic, nagging fear of being caught. It is better that corrections be made when there is less to lose.

Discovery of significantly misrepresented or falsified credentials should cause the professional association to take disciplinary action, even to the point of expulsion. Representation of a fictitious academic degree or position is significant both to the employer and the professional organization.

Slovenly verification by potential employers contributes to the ease with which false or exaggerated credentials are used. This is true even of candidates for senior management positions. The employer is responsible for adequately checking credentials and taking action as necessary when dishonesty is uncovered.

Employers have an obligation to report performance of former employees accurately. In the case of serious problems, such as a drug addiction, specific information should be reported, whether or not it was requested. For less serious problems, a fair and balanced appraisal that reports strengths as well as weaknesses meets ethical obligations.[6]

A Massachusetts case raised questions about ethical behavior when physicians writing references neglected to include information relevant to understanding the character of former residents in anesthesiology.

But Is It Relevant?

The Massachusetts Medical Society plans to investigate three doctors at a major Boston hospital who wrote highly laudatory letters recommending a colleague only a few days after he had been sentenced to jail for raping a nurse.

The convicted physician . . . was able to use the letters to get a new job as an anesthesiologist at the Children's Hospital in Buffalo, where officials said they were unaware of his legal troubles. [He] . . . was charged last week in another Boston rape case, in 1978, involving patients.

Medical officials say the case, involving doctors at the Brigham and Women's Hospital here, is the most striking example they have encountered of how letters of recommendation for hospital jobs have lost their value in recent years, as physicians became cautious about writing anything critical about colleagues for fear of being sued.

. . . Other doctors on the staff of the hospital said they believed the letters were written after . . . consulting with the attorney for the Brigham and Women's Hospital. Since the rape did not occur within the hospital, they suggested that the attorney had advised the doctors that they had no basis for being critical of [the physician's] medical performance.

B. J. Anderson, associate general counsel for the American Medical Association, . . . said that the association advised directors of departments in hospitals to be candid when writing letters of recommendations despite the threat of lawsuits. But, Mr. Anderson said, "Too frequently hospitals that have had a problem with a doctor will write a glowing letter because it is easier to export your problems across a state line than to resolve them yourself."[7]

The Massachusetts Medical Society investigated the conduct of the doctors who wrote the letters of recommendation. All three were censured and put on a year's probation. The controversy over the letters prompted appointment of a panel to suggest guidelines for preparing letters of recommendation. Its report advised physicians to follow a Golden Rule of letter writing. This means "that a letter should contain the information known to the writer which he would like to have were he to receive the letter." The report went on to say that "information regarding personal character is of great importance in the case of physicians."[8]

Whether or not the doctors who wrote the letters of recommendations violated the letter of the law, they certainly failed to honor its spirit. Any health services organization that might hire these physicians would find it relevant that they had been convicted of a crime. This is especially true of a crime such as rape, which involves moral turpitude. As with nonphysician staff and employees, the organization has a moral obligation to report relevant information about physicians honestly amd objectively.

ALLOCATING RESOURCES

Ethical issues are raised as managers make resource allocation decisions. Whether resource allocation affects populations or groups (macroallocation) or individuals (microallocation), allocation involves making choices. Decision making is based on explicit or implicit criteria. Some managers use subjective judgments about social worth, usefulness to society, and need. Other managers use more objective criteria: use of a lottery or a queue, or ability to pay. Values and philosophical statements about individuals and society underlie both, even though these are usually implicit and may be only vaguely understood by decision makers.

Various methods and guidelines are used by decision makers in allocating resources. Decisions made by governments are often based on economic motives or political effect. Like governments, health services organizations involve managers and clinicians in macroallocation decisions. Microallocation involves decision making about clinical treatment for individuals, and involves nonclinician managers to a much lesser degree. Important aspects of microallocation decision making are a physician's willingness to refer, patient access to services and technologies and their applications, and economic considerations. Micro decision making is often guided (in a sense, prejudged) by macroallocation policies that the organization (or government) has adopted.

As discussed in Chapter 1, utilitarians judge the morality of an act by assessing the results produced and determining if the greatest good for the greatest number is achieved. Economists and managers use this approach in their cost–benefit analyses. Applying criteria of utility is only a partial answer, however. This narrow approach ignores considerations of human need, fairness, and justice, all of which health services managers find important.

Macroallocation

Specific theories have been developed to suggest how macroallocation does or should occur. The concept of a right to health care is prominent in several theories. At one extreme is a theory that asserts that all technologies should be available to all persons. A corollary to this hyperegalitarian position is that if technology is not available to all, it should be available to none. This theory is based on respect for persons, which mandates that society recognize every person's inherent right to receive health services. To some, providing different levels of treatment implies that some persons are, in effect, paid less respect than others. Equal respect means receiving equal levels of services. Absent this, the service should not be available to any.

At the other end of the continuum are those who argue that access to health services is not a right guaranteed by society, but a privilege. This hyperindividualistic position also holds that health services providers, such as physicians, have no obligation to render services. In providing services, health care providers act out of free will and humanitarian instinct. The hyperindividualists argue that if there is a right to health care, providers then have an obligation to render services. This duty to render services diminishes the freedom and dignity of providers, and fails to recognize their value and worth as human beings, thus violating the respect they are owed.

Between these extremes is the position that society has a duty to assist in developing, encouraging, and even providing health services. Fried suggests that routine basic services ought to be available to all (what he calls the "decent minimum"). More exotic high-technology services are limited in a number of ways (e.g., location, cost, referrals) and must be available on a different basis.[9] Where to draw this line is a political decision, and depends on society's willingness to provide the resources needed.

Health services managers face similar macroallocation questions; the principles are almost identical to those applied by government decision makers. Questions of who gets what, when, where, and how are found in many issues faced by health services managers—whether to build a new outpatient department, when to purchase an MRI machine, and how to allocate staff. Increasingly, answers to these questions require close attention to economic considerations. Financial well-being is critical, since it enables the organization to engage in its mission, one aspect of which is service to the socially and economically disadvantaged.

The Feasibility of BEAM

Brain electrical activity mapping (BEAM) is a recently developed technology to image the brain. It significantly improves the physician's ability to localize an abnormality. In response to increased demands for the procedure from staff radiologists and local neurologists and reports in the literature on the usefulness of BEAM testing, Metropolitan Hospital decided to investigate the possibility of acquiring access to it. The options include: contracting for use of a BEAM machine, purchasing a BEAM machine, and approaching neighboring County Hospital about sharing its recently acquired BEAM machine.

One of the factors in this decision is uncertainty as to how changes in reimbursement will affect hospital revenues. Because of this concern and the fact that all options involve a major expenditure of capital funds, the chairman asked the CEO to form a committee to evaluate all options, including foregoing access to BEAM testing. This assessment will be used to make a final decision between BEAM and a proposed addition to the intensive care unit (ICU), a project that has strong support from the surgical staff and that has already been delayed twice.

The board would like to delay this decision until the reimbursement implications are understood, but several attending physicians have stated that BEAM testing is critical to their practices. They have stated that although they prefer the nursing staff at Metropolitan, they will be forced to admit certain patients to County in order to use BEAM. A rumor has just surfaced among the medical staff that several prominent members are considering forming a consortium to purchase and operate BEAM and other diagnostic equipment in a professional office complex under construction. [10]

What are the important aspects of this case? First, the new technology will improve the quality of care. Second, its availability will affect the organization's financial situation—operating costs are high, typically exceeding capital costs within a few years. Financial considerations are complicated by the new prospective payment system. Third, the medical staff is divided about the expenditure, and this adds to the complexity of medical staff politics. Fourth, BEAM is expensive technology. This makes the decision even more important and difficult.

The obvious starting point in solving this problem is to review the organizational philosophy and mission. If Metropolitan Hospital has a mission of serving special populations or needs, both BEAM and an ICU addition may use resources in a manner consistent with that mission. Are there even better uses for the resources? The considerations raised above are not easily addressed, but internal decision processes, such as an ethics committee, provide a means of solving the problem of BEAM. The expected context for decision making will be the organizational philosophy, as reflected in the strategic plan. These were described in Chapter 5. The technological imperative is present not only in delivering services to individual patients, but in macroallocation decisions as well.

Microallocation

One usually thinks of microallocation decisions in terms of exotic life-saving treatment (ELST). All scarce resources require allocation, however.

Who Gets the Penicillin?

In 1943, penicillin was in short supply among U.S. armed forces in North Africa. Competitors for its use were two groups of soldiers suffering from infections that would respond to it: soldiers with venereal disease and soldiers with battle wounds. The chief surgical consultant advised that priority be given to the wounded; the theatre medical commander directed that priority be given to soldiers with venereal disease, arguing that soldiers cured of venereal disease could be restored to fighting trim more rapidly, and that left untreated, such men represented a threat of spreading the infection to others. The decision to use the penicillin on the soldiers with venereal disease represented a very pragmatic judgment in accord with the morality of social utility in a situation in which objectives—achievement of maximum fighting power as rapidly as possible—were narrowly defined. For better or worse, life is rarely so circumscribed in its goals. [11]

Treating only the men infected with venereal disease is the morally correct choice only if the utilitarian criterion of returning the greatest number of men to the line as quickly as possible is applied. This decision is made without judging the relative worth of the soldiers in need of treatment or the means by which they came to require treatment.

Foreign transplant recipients obtaining organs such as kidneys from American donors suggests another dimension of microallocation decisions. These patients tend to come from countries in which technological impediments or religious customs prevent organ harvesting. They are health services consumers who pay with their own resources rather than through insurance or government programs. In that regard, they are favored by transplant centers. In addition, they are generally willing to accept organs that may be somewhat older or do not present optimal tissue matches. The transplanting of American organs in foreigners raises legitimate concern about priorities in a system in which American patients wait for organs while non-Americans receive them.

Theories of allocating ELST to individual patients have been developed by Childress and Rescher. [12] They address the problem of how decisions about who gets what should be made. Childress rejects considerations of subjective criteria, such as worth to society, because such comparisons demean the potential recipient and run counter to the belief in the inherent dignity of each human being. His position is Kantian, because it stresses respect for persons and its derivative, autonomy. He argues that a system that views all persons needing treatment as equals recognizes inherent human worth. Once medical criteria are used to determine the need and appropriateness of therapy, opportunities for ELST should be available on a first come, first served basis, or alternatively, through some random selection process, such as a lottery.

A leading ethicist, the late Paul Ramsey, agreed with Childress as to the desirability of a lottery, or a policy of first come, first served that ignores the subjective judgments one finds in other, criteria-oriented schemes. At the same time, Ramsey found nondiscriminatory predetermined and announced rules based on statistical medical probabilities acceptable. This view would, for example, permit groups such as the very young and the very old to be excluded from dialysis programs.[13]

Rescher's schema is two tiered. The first tier is devoted to basic screening, and applies to groups of potential patients. It consists of factors such as constituency served, benefit to science, and likelihood of success by type of treatment or recipient. The second tier deals with individuals. It judges medical factors (e.g., relative likelihood of success, life expectancy) and social aspects, such as family role, potential future contributions, and past services rendered. Rescher concludes by saying that if all factors are equal, a random selection process should be used for the final choice. For Rescher, the social aspects cause the most difficulty because they are heavily dependent on value judgments. However, he considers it irrational to make choices subject to chance, even if medical criteria are objective.

Each of these theories of microallocation has advantages and disadvantages, both morally and pragmatically. Each develops a formal or semiformal process that permits users to address issues and problems in an organized fashion. While these approaches may not make possible a decision that satisfies everyone, the theories offer the advantage of an identified system that at least provides frameworks within which to make decisions. Given particular medical criteria, an individual's chances of being selected for medical services may be unpredictable (Childress), partially predictable (Ramsey), or almost totally predictable (Rescher). The basis for selection may hinge on largely subjective criteria (Rescher), or may be solely a matter of chance and in that sense eminently fair to all who need the treatment (Childress), or who meet the criteria for medical statistical probabilities (Ramsey).

Choices

Randy Glenn had just fallen asleep when the phone rang. It was the night supervisor at the comprehensive care center and hospital of which Glenn was the CEO. The supervisor was quite agitated and had trouble getting her words out. It took a few minutes for the message to become clear. One of Glenn's nightmares had come true: the four-bed ICU was full and an emergency case had just come in.

The new patient had been injured in a car accident. She was stabilized in the emergency department, but neither air medevac nor mobile ICU ambulance services were available. It is certain that she would not survive being transferred by any other means. She had to get into the ICU within 2 hours.

The night supervisor recovered somewhat and quickly described the patients currently occupying ICU beds:

Patient A: 60-year-old female, comatose, stroke victim who required respirator support; 27 days in the ICU; uncertain prognosis; retired; no family; city resident

Patient B: 9-year-old Down syndrome male with acute respiratory infection; 4 days in ICU; family in adjacent city

Patient C: 36-year-old male who had undergone an emergency appendectomy, developed severe wound infection and probable septicemia; source of infection unknown; requires ICU care for blood pressure instability secondary to sepsis; bachelor; elderly mother lives in city

Patient D: 12-year-old female; undergoing chemotherapy for leukemia with an experimental drug; had been in remission three times; monitoring of experimental protocol and potential reaction to drug requires ICU care, family in city

New Patient: 24-year-old female; college honor student in physics, scholarship winner; pregnant; engaged; no family known

The supervisor ended by asking, "What should I do?" Indeed, what to do, thought Glenn, who wished the institutional ethics committee had been more active. Glenn pondered the alternatives as the garage door opened and the 10-minute trip to the hospital began.[14]

This is the classic "last bed in the ICU" situation. Under Childress's and Ramsey's criteria, if all patients are assumed equally in need of ICU care, the new patient would be left to receive the best care she could get outside the ICU. Applying Rescher's criteria, the prognosis for one of the current patients is not as good as the prognosis for the new patient. Thus, one of the existing patients should be removed from the ICU. None of the models permits patients unable to get ICU care to be abandoned and left to fend for themselves. In all of the approaches, they would receive the best alternative care the facility could offer.

Public awareness of how choices are made may or may not enhance the public's view that health services organizations and the system act in a just manner. But public scrutiny will cause greater attention to decision criteria, the decision process, and the fairness of their application. Kantian principles of respect for persons and not using persons as ends are reflected in Childress's approach, which stresses autonomy. Rescher includes a mix of Kantian and utilitarian views and, most importantly, emphasizes justice, as described in Chapter 1. Currently, few health services organizations determine resource allocation within the context of formally recognized ethical criteria. As with macroallocation decisions, these criteria must be developed within the context of the organizational philosophy and mission statement.

CONCLUSION

This chapter identifies and analyzes ethical problems managers face in dealing with confidential information. Managers' relationships with governing bodies and medical staffs are identified within an ethical context, as are some of the implications of falsified or overstated personal qualifications.

Attention is also paid to macro- and microallocation of resources. Questions related to the allocation of resources are common to all types of health services organizations, but are often not recognized. Both macro- and microallocation issues are becoming more important as resource constraints increase, and it is crucial that the organizational philosophy and mission statement provide guidance for these decisions. This guidance requires a level of precision and specificity in philosophy and mission that many health services organizations currently lack. This deficit must be overcome.

NOTES

1. See, for example, Charles U. Letourneau, *Hospital Trusteeship* (Chicago: Sterling Publications, 1959), 90–91; Charles U. Letourneau, *The Hospital Administrator* (Chicago: Sterling Publications, 1969), 45; and Malcolm T. MacEachern, *Hospital Organization and Management* (Berwyn, IL: Physicians' Record Co., 1962), 87, 97.

2. Peter A. Weil and Stuart A. Wesbury, Jr., "The Shifting Roles of CEOs and Trustees," *Trustee 37*, no. 7 (July 1984): 26.

3. James D. Harvey, "Evaluating the Performance of the Chief Executive Officer," *Hospital & Health Services Administration 23* (Spring 1978): 5–21.

4. Daniel R. Longo, Jeffrey Alexander, Paul Earle, and Marni Pahl, "Profile of Hospital Governance: A Report from the Nation's Hospitals," *Trustee 43*, no. 5 (May 1990): 7.

5. Rockwell Schulz and Alton C. Johnson, *Management of Hospitals*, 2nd ed. (New York: McGraw-Hill, 1983), 160–161.

6. Bonnie J. Gray and Robert K. Landrum, "Difficulties With Being Ethical," *Business 33* (July–September 1983): 32.

7. Fox Butterfield, "Doctors' Praise Assailed for Peer in Rape Case," *New York Times,* September 24, 1981.

8. "Doctors Censured in Massachusetts," *New York Times,* February 4, 1982.

9. Charles Fried, "Equality and Rights in Medical Care," *Hastings Center Report 6* (February 1976): 29–34.

10. Adapted from Jonathon S. Rakich, Beaufort B. Longest, Jr., and Kurt Darr, *Managing Health Services Organizations,* 2nd. ed., (Philadelphia: W. B. Saunders, 1985), 141. Used with permission.

11. Ibid., 139–140. Used with permission.

12. James F. Childress, "Who Shall Live When Not All Can Live?" *Soundings, An Interdisciplinary Journal 53*, no. 4 (Winter 1970): 339–355; Nicholas Rescher, "The Allocation of Exotic Medical Lifesaving Therapy," *Ethics 79*, no. 3 (April 1969): 173–186.

13. Paul Ramsey, *The Patient as Person* (New Haven: Yale University Press, 1970), 252.

14. Adapted from Jonathon S. Rakich, Beaufort B. Longest, Jr., and Kurt Darr, *Managing Health Services Organizations,* 2nd ed. (Philadelphia: W. B. Saunders, 1985), 139–140. Used with permission.

8

∞

ETHICAL DUTIES TOWARD PATIENTS AND COMMUNITY

THIS CHAPTER IDENTIFIES THE SPECIAL relationships between managers (and their organizations) and patients and the community. Duties and obligations managers have toward themselves and toward their profession were noted earlier within the context of the moral philosophies and the ethical principles of respect for persons, beneficence, nonmaleficence, and justice. That discussion highlighted the need for managers to have a personal ethic to guide their decision making on administrative and biomedical ethical problems within the context of the organizational philosophy. The book's underlying premise that the manager is a moral agent with independent duties to the patient is reinforced in this chapter. Managers must juxtapose their relationship with and duty of loyalty toward the organization with their relationships with patients. Reciprocal duties among colleagues are part of being in a professional group that has expectations and demands certain behavior. In many ways the organization is the manager. Managers must keep this in mind, because their actions and decisions are judged in that context. There are, however, ethical limits to what the organization has a right to expect of persons working for or affiliated with it. Managers must know the limits of their personal ethic and must speak out when the organization infringes on it.

ORGANIZATIONAL CONTEXT OF RELATIONSHIPS

The manager is employed as an agent of the governing body to carry out the organization's mission within the context of its philosophy. This relationship is most apparent in the activities of the CEO. It is no less true, however, for subordinate managers. Regardless of their level in the organization, managers must keep in mind that they are moral agents, and are not excused from the effects of their actions because they are employees or are following orders. Managers are accountable for their actions and their effects on patients, colleagues, and the organization. While the law and its enforcement may excuse those who are not prime actors or decision makers, managers remain responsible for their actions morally.

As an employee, the manager has a duty of loyalty to the organization and its staff. This duty of loyalty means that the manager supports the employer's goals and activities. Disagreements about policy or policy implementation are not broadcast about or shared with persons who have no need to know. This duty of loyalty is especially important in light of a common malady, backbiting the employer. Backbiting does not refer to the grumbling or complaining that is considered healthy and normal behavior. Although employees may have a legitimate reason to complain about treatment they have received—not even the best employer does things right every time—rabid comments are problematic in an organization. Employees who persistently badmouth their employer are behaving unacceptably, and should find new employment, voluntarily or involuntarily.

Managers must achieve the difficult balance between loyalty to the organization and faithfulness to their personal ethic and professional integrity. Where does the manager draw the line? How far should a manager go in following the crowd, or in standing alone? A clear baseline is needed to answer questions like these. It is here that the manager's personal ethic is crucial. Professional codes of ethics play a role, but they provide only general guidance, and are unlikely to be useful in helping a manager decide what to do in specific cases. At the extreme, the question of loyalty is part of whistleblowing, which is examined later in this chapter.

As posited earlier, the manager has an independent duty and responsibility toward the patient. At a minimum, this means that managers must protect patients and help further their interests. What follows from that is the need for integrity and the courage to speak out and act to make that responsibility a reality.

All He Had to Do Was Ask

Richard Weidner experienced angina on mild exercise. His internist referred him to University Hospital for a cardiac catheterization. Weidner was pleased to have had a long, friendly visit with the cardiologist, who had assured him that she would be performing the procedure on him.

That afternoon, Weidner was lying on the table ready for the catheterization to start. He had a clear view of the television monitor showing the catheter being threaded from his groin to his heart. At one point he asked what was happening and was surprised when the cardiologist appeared near his head and described the procedure. When Weidner asked her who was actually threading the catheter, he was told it was a resident in cardiology.

Later, Weidner was in a recovery area, waiting to be discharged. He was quite agitated about the fact that a resident had performed the procedure, especially since he had thought he had an understanding with the cardiologist. He described the situation to the nurse, and demanded she explain how the doctor could have done such a thing. The nurse said, "You know, this is a teaching hospital and we have to help train residents to perform these procedures." Weidner wasn't placated. He said, "I probably would have let the resident participate if I had been asked. But, they didn't ask me, and I'm damned angry about it. Please ask one of the managers to come see me, I want some answers."

Weidner was not harmed—at least not physically—nor was his action motivated by malicious intent. The basic issue may be the insensitivity of the hospital and the fact that its teaching program conflicts with the patient's role and voice. Clearly lacking here is respect for the patient. The staff (including the cardiologist and resident) were likely following normal procedure. They would probably be upset to learn that one of their patients was angry about how he had been treated. To become fully qualified physicians, residents need specialized training, which can be gained only by treating patients. What is far less acceptable, of course, is the assumption that patients are automatically willing to participate. Being used as a means to an end is a utilitarian view, one that is incompatible with the principle of respect for persons (specifically, autonomy).

Teaching hospitals usually include general disclosures about the organization's teaching activities on their admission forms. By signing these forms, patients agree to participate in teaching activities. Few patients, however, take the time to read and understand this information. Judged by reasonable standards of informed consent, signing this form has little validity. Even assuming the form has been read and understood, it is common courtesy to inform the patient when teaching activities are actually taking place, and to ask specific permission then. To do so meets minimum requirements of ethical conduct. (Medical education and consent are considered again in Chapter 9.)

In this case, Weidner was actively misled. The identity of the physician who would do the procedure was of sufficient concern to him that he sought reassurance from someone in a position of trust. This brought an inaccurate response from the cardiologist. What should the manager of cardiology do when Weidner tells his story? Except to reassure and placate, there is little that can be done. More important is what should be done about future events like this one. A personal ethic (and organizational philosophy) should make it clear that efforts will be made to prevent repetition. Basic changes may be necessary to convince physicians and employed clinical staff that their interactions with patients are to be based on respect for persons. This means that more attention must be paid to seeking permission and communicating with patients.

MONITORING CLINICAL ACTIVITIES

Managers act for the organization. But as decision makers whose actions have moral implications and as members of a profession, managers are never simply instruments of the organization. Managers have a duty to patients that is independent of the duty of the organization toward the patient, or the duty of the physician toward the patient. This duty is not limited to problems with the business office or the quality of food, but extends to clinical activities. In terms of the patient, the manager is the organization's conscience.

Nonphysician managers do not judge clinical activities as a physican would. Just as they use technical experts to develop a new computer system or prepare a loss prevention management program, managers rely on clinical experts in nursing and medicine to assist in understanding these services and their results. As managers gain experience in health services, their enhanced knowledge about the clinical aspects increasingly enables them to determine when problems are present. Even though they may become quite sophisticated, their purpose is not to serve as junior physicians, but to understand what physicians do and what they need and want. The primary reason to understand clinical activities is to help the organization serve patients.

This involvement works both ways, and managers should expect and seek physician involvement in administrative decision making. The evidence suggests that hospitals in which physicians participate in management decision making are more efficient and effective.

An important role of managers in clinical settings is to act as a link between the formal and informal organizations. Anecdotal evidence about quality assurance makes it clear that informal communications are useful (perhaps even critical) in identifying clinical problems, and serve as an important supplement to formal systems. Nursing is especially important as an informal link. Deficient performance by physicians is often first identified by the nurses who work with them. Information provided by nurses or others can put the formal system on alert, and be a starting point for further inquiry. No action can be based on rumor, however; it is incumbent upon the manager that there be adequate follow-up and investigation, preferably in conjunction with normal quality assurance activities. Should it be necessary, however, the manager must take the independent action needed to protect the patient. As a moral agent, the prudent, ethical manager cannot ignore situations that jeopardize the patient or the organization.

A Different Kind of Risk

Dr. Sagatius has just returned to his office after seeing the risk manager. He was very upset and slammed the door behind him before slumping into his chair. He wouldn't stand for it, not again, he said to himself. This was the final straw. Hospital administration wasn't going to push him around.

He thought back to the previous two incidents in the pediatrics unit, and remarked to himself how similar they were. Now a third incident had transpired. He had complained to the nursing director when the other two medication errors had been committed by the same nurse. Now it appeared he would have to go higher.

Another one of his patients had been medicated incorrectly—actually overdosed. Fortunately, Dr. Sagatius had been able to intervene before serious consequences, probably even death, occurred. Nonetheless, the child would have to stay in the hospital for at least a week longer, and one couldn't be sure whether there might be longer-lasting consequences.

The day after the last incident, Dr. Sagatius had been asked by the risk manager to stop by her office to discuss what had happened. While he was there, he noticed that the risk manager had the child's medical record on the desk. Dr. Sagatius noticed that the risk manager had changed the medication record; he knew it had previously shown the overdose. When he asked her about it, she said it really didn't matter because there was no apparent harm to the child. "Why needlessly upset the parents?" she asked. When Dr. Sagatius protested that this wasn't honest, the risk manager became hostile and reminded Dr. Sagatius that a malpractice suit would hurt all those affiliated with the hospital, including the doctors, who were almost certain to be sued should this error come to light. She warned him not to discuss the problem with the parents. Dr. Sagatius had planned to tell the parents what had happened, believing that they were owed an explanation for the extra days in the hospital and that they also should be aware of the need to watch for certain telltale signs of the overdose that might show up in the future.

Dr. Sagatius weighed the various possibilities. He knew he had to tell the parents to watch the child very closely, even if he didn't discuss the overdose. He went to get the parents' telephone number.

Dr. Sagatius faces two ethical problems. The first concerns the risk manager. Ethically, Dr. Sagatius's primary duty is to protect the interests of his patient. This necessitates giving the parents whatever information they need to assist in caring for the child. Providing this information is consistent with the principles of beneficence and nonmaleficence. How can he carry out this duty given the position of the risk manager? The risk manager has violated the principle of respect for persons. In addition, by being willing to cover up clinical failures she is perpetuating a system that violates the principle of nonmaleficence.

The second ethical problem involves the director of nursing, who has not taken steps to prevent a serious problem in the pediatrics unit, a problem that has occurred on three occasions. Such inaction is inconsistent with the principles of beneficence and nonmaleficence.

Falsifying the medical record is not common, but it is common for the organization to submerge its ethical obligations into the legal aspects of a case, and to treat the patient as an enemy. There is a strong tendency to want to cover up failure. Patients and family often sense this. Not only is such behavior likely to spur them to press even harder for an explanation, but it makes it more likely that they will sue as a way to vent their anger. This utilitarian argument also supports taking the unpleasant but preferred step of being forthright and honest with patients who have been injured. Anecdotal evidence suggests that patients and families can understand that mistakes occur and things do go wrong. Organizations that acknowledge this fact and do all they can to make things right are much better served than those that circle the wagons and make a last-ditch stand.

Scrutiny of health services delivery by all members of the organization, especially managers, and taking action as necessary should not be seen by any of the parties involved as "ratting" or being a stool pigeon. Such an interpretation can be made only if one ignores the reason for being of the organization and those who work there. It, and they, are there to further the interests of the patient. When there are problems in the delivery of services, the organization and its managers must act to minimize loss and injury to the patient and do what is reasonably necessary to make the patient whole. The manager must be involved, as necessary, to eliminate or reduce recurrence of problems in clinical services.

WHISTLEBLOWING

When an employee reveals information about illegal, inefficient, or wasteful action that endangers the health, safety, or freedom of the public it is called *whistleblowing*.[1] This definition is broad enough to include revelation of mismanagement. As used here, whistleblowing includes the disclosure of information both within the organization and externally.

Whistleblowing affects virtually all sectors of public and private enterprise.[2] Three types of activities are affected by whistleblowing: clear illegality, potential illegality or danger, and business social policy.[3] Clear illegality occurs when the law is knowingly violated. Examples include falsifying test results reported to government agencies, bribing government inspectors, making illegal campaign contributions, falsifying audit reports, deliberately violating labor laws, discriminating by race or sex in employment, and deliberately dumping dangerous wastes inappropriately.[4]

The second type of whistleblowing involves potential illegality or danger. A growing body of regulation and case law protects worker health, patient safety, public health, and the environment. In addition, managers and employees are moral agents, who are morally obligated to take action when there is reason to believe that patients are at risk, regardless of other requirements. In most situations in which whistleblowing occurs or should occur, the whistleblower acts in the belief that a given practice, process, or result is either not in compliance with accepted standards or places the patient unnecessarily at risk.

"In any well-run enterprise, management should be seriously concerned about such violations and should welcome warnings by its own employees . . . ."[5]

The third type of whistleblowing involves the organization's social policy. An employee may become concerned about the morality of a management policy and its effect on patients or society. An example from Chapter 11 is that of an employee who is opposed to abortion and sterilization. Speaking out or refusing to participate is likely to be protected by conscience clauses in state or federal statute or by the Constitution, if state action is involved. Assuming the policy is legal, employee protest raises two issues: the empoyee's right to free speech and the employee's responsibility as a moral agent. Employees are entitled to the same constitutionally protected right of free speech as other persons. Furthermore, as moral agents they have an ethical duty to speak out when policies and actions could or do adversely affect patients or society. The controversy typically arises when an employee exercises the right of free speech or the duty of moral agency by speaking publicly against a lawful organizational policy and thereby harms the organization's reputation and market advantage.[6]

Place of Whistleblowing

Leading commercial companies have created ombudsman programs in which a single individual receives, investigates, and responds to employee complaints. Such programs are important for employees who believe illegal or improper conduct is occurring. The problem with using an ombudsman is that the ombudsman may lack the authority to solve problems in line departments. The ombudsman may not be empowered to deal with senior managers who actively promote illegal or improper conduct as an organizational imperative.[7]

Even where employees are protected by law, as in federal employment, they continue to fear reprisals. A 1983 survey by the Merit Systems Protection Board found that 69% of workers who said they knew firsthand of some example of government waste failed to report it. The most common reason cited was a belief that nothing would be done about the problem; fear of reprisal was a close second. This fear was borne out by the fact that 23% of workers who said they had publicly reported a case of fraud also claimed to have suffered reprisals through demotion, poor performance ratings, or losing a promotion. Those who continued reporting problems did so anonymously.[8]

It is crucial that there be a change in the current health services organization concepts, which is typically an "I win, you lose" (zero-sum) approach to whistleblowing. Responsible reporting can be used to benefit employees and employers. "Directing corrective efforts to (whistleblowers) instead of the policy or practice they protest will not alter the conditions that make whistleblowing necessary."[9]

The concept of moral agency and the willingness to speak and act, as necessary, remain central, recurring themes for managers and caregivers alike.

> The issue of professional dissent is critical, not only to the field of health services administration, but to the delivery of health services. There is no morality without action; ethics cannot survive unless people speak their consciences when it really matters. . . . One distinguishing mark of professionals is the ability to recognize ethical problems, (and) to act as moral custodians of the organization in which they work. . . .[10]

In 1986, a significant new dimension was added to whistleblowing when Congress enacted a law, the False Claims Act, that strengthened protection for individuals who discovered and reported fraud in federally funded programs. One provision allows them to sue in the name of the federal government, with the incentive that they will receive 15%–30% of any triple damages and fines that are imposed. Such suits are known as *qui tam* actions, from the Latin phrase "who as well for the king for himself sues in the matter." The vast amounts of money spent by the federal government in programs such as Medicare means that the potential for fraud in health services is great. It is likely that many *qui tam* suits will be brought against health services organizations, especially hospitals. Such efforts to identify and deal with fraud may help the organization and its managers understand what is acceptable practice and modify their performance accordingly.

Examples of Whistleblowing

The health services system and individual health services organizations face a dilemma when they encourage employees to act responsibly in all situations without causing unnecessary disruption. This dilemma will be even more difficult to resolve as organizations become more competitive. Employees will be asked to deal aggressively with external competitors, but will be expected to be complacent internally.

How Sweet It Is!

Dr. A. Grace Pierce joined the research staff of Ortho Pharmaceutical Corporation in 1971. In 1975, she was part of a team developing a prescription drug known generically as loperamide. The drug was used to treat acute and chronic diarrhea in infants, children, and the elderly. Saccharin was used to make it palatable by masking its bitter taste.

The research team agreed that the formula was unsuitable because it substantially exceeded FDA limits of saccharin. Management was informed of this fact, but nevertheless decided to file a new drug application with the FDA. Other members of the research team decided to continue development, but Dr. Pierce refused. Although she was offered work in other projects at no decrease in pay, she resigned her position, apparently believing her refusal had irrevocably damaged her career at Ortho.

Later, she sought relief in the courts, alleging wrongful

discharge. The New Jersey Supreme Court ruled that Ortho had not acted illegally and that there were no grounds for a cause of action.[11]

The court put substantial weight on the fact that harm to the public was not imminent. The Court ruled that the ethic of the Hippocratic Oath did not contain a clear mandate of public policy that would have prevented Dr. Pierce from continuing her research.

Similar cases have been set in health services organizations.

It's Really Only an X-Ray

Frances O'Sullivan was an X-ray technician employed by several radiologists and a hospital. She brought suit for breach of an employment contract after she was fired. She alleged she was fired for refusal to perform catheterizations, a procedure she had not been trained to perform. O'Sullivan could not legally perform catheterizations in New Jersey, where only licensed nurses and physicians may do so. The issue involved was unique in that the plaintiff had been asked to perform an illegal act. The superior court denied the defendant physicians' and hospital's motion to dismiss.[12]

Denying the motion to dismiss meant that O'Sullivan was entitled to a trial. Since there is no report this occurred, it may be assumed that the case was settled out of court. In light of the illegality of the act, O'Sullivan clearly acted properly.

Another actual case is also illustrative.

Don't Speak Now and Forever Hold Your Peace

Linda Rafferty was a psychiatric nurse at a state institution, where she was appalled by conditions. The abuses Rafferty claimed to have observed included the staff's failure to protect patients from homosexual abuse by other patients and from sexual exploitation by outside workmen; improper nonpsychiatric medical care; allowing patients to keep medications in their rooms; locking up fire extinguishers; leaving blank prescription forms, signed in advance by physicians, in unlocked drawers for nurses to fill out on weekends; and chronic absenteeism on the part of hospital medical staff. Rafferty repeatedly complained to her superiors, but resigned when her protests brought no change.

She was hired at another institution, Community Mental Health Center, as supervisor of nurses. Before she was hired, she gave an interview to a Philadelphia newspaper in which she was sharply critical of treatment at the state institution. The morning after the story appeared, she was fired from her new position because "staff members were upset about the article." No other reasons were given until trial, when the Health Center alleged inadequate job performance as well.

Rafferty brought suit alleging she had been deprived of her constitutional rights. The court ruled that she be reinstated and awarded over $3,000 in back pay.[13]

These cases highlight the three significant issues relating to whistleblowing as an ethical problem in health services organizations. The first is employee responsibility and accountability, something that applies to all employees, whether or not they are managers. The second issue is fair practices. To encourage responsibility and accountability, due process procedures are necessary to protect employees who consider themselves moral agents and are courageous enough to speak out. Due process regarding employee disciplinary actions (both in terms of procedure and substance) is necessary, whether or not the organization is one to which federal or state constitutional protections apply. Being bound by such requirements will also encourage others to act when they should. Methods must be developed to balance the individual's duty toward the employer against the duty toward the public. This can be difficult. As has been pointed out, ". . . many of the rights and privileges . . . so important to a free society that they are constitutionally protected . . . are vulnerable to abuse through an employer's power."[14] The third issue is how the organization can encourage employees to speak out in appropriate ways to carry out their independent duty toward the patient, without causing unnecessary damage to the indispensable cooperative and trust relationships that exist inside health services organizations, as well as between such organizations and their communities.

Negative Aspects of Whistleblowing

Positive aspects of whistleblowing are tempered by several negative aspects:

1. Not all whistleblowers are correct in what they allege to be the facts of management's misconduct. Determining the accuracy of whistleblowing charges is not always easy.
2. There is always the danger that incompetent or inadequate employees will become whistleblowers to avoid facing justifiable personnel sanctions.
3. Employees can whistleblow in ways that are unacceptably disruptive, regardless of the merits of their protest.
4. Some whistleblowers are not protesting unlawful or unsafe behavior but social policies by management that the employee considers unwise or unethical.
5. The legal definitions of what constitutes a safe product, danger to health, or improper treatment of employees are often not clear.
6. The efficiency and flexibility of personnel administration could be threatened by the creation of legal rights to dissent and legalized review systems.

7. There can be risks to the desirable autonomy of the private sector because review of allegations by whistleblowers will expand government too deeply into internal business policies.[15]

Creation of an ongoing attitude of responsibility, openness, and commitment on the part of top management is the first step in developing a meaningful internal policy on whistleblowing. The next step is drafting the principles and policy statements that apply management's intention throughout the organization and communicating the policy to employees. The importance of middle and line managers must be stressed. Not only must they be knowledgeable about the policy, but reviews must ensure their adherence to it.[16]

KEEPING BYLAWS CURRENT AND ENFORCING ADMINISTRATIVE PROVISIONS

Other important responsibilities of senior management are to help the medical staff keep its bylaws current and to assist in enforcing administrative provisions. A typical example of the latter occurs when the CEO or chief operating officer applies the medical staff bylaws, and the rules and regulations as they require suspension of a physician's admitting privileges. This commonly occurs because the medical records of that physician's patients are not current. Actions such as these are not taken singlehandedly (absent an emergency situation), but are made through preestablished procedures and channels. Because of the independent duty owed the patient, even exclusively clinical problems cannot be ignored by managers. When there is evidence of a need to act, the manager must do so.

Neither administrative nor clinical problems can be solved by ignoring them. Once known, problems can be covered up for a time, but, as Watergate demonstrated, they are eventually brought to light. A normal reaction to revelations of scandals or major problems in an organization is that others, perhaps many people, must have known. How could the situation have occurred or been allowed to continue? In addition to the moral guidelines of respect for persons and the need for honesty in all interactions, the likelihood of discovery is a utilitarian reason for recognizing and solving problems early.

EVALUATING PERSONNEL

Organized efforts to ensure that all clinical practitioners are qualified and practice at an acceptable level protects patients and furthers their interests in the health services system. Qualifications of health providers are determined on initial application to the organization. Periodic reviews ensure that medical staff remain qualified. While this process applies to all who render clinical care, most attention is given to the medical staff. Preventing legal actions and bad publicity are not unimportant, but the primary reasons to be concerned about competence are respect for the principles of beneficence, aiding the patient, and nonmaleficence.

Beginning in January, 1985, the Joint Commission on Accreditation of Healthcare Organizations (JCAHO) permitted nonphysician and nondentist independent allied health professionals (IAHPs) to serve as members of the medical staff. IAHPs are licensed to deliver a limited range of health services, and include providers such as nurse midwives and clinical psychologists. Previously, JCAHO did not allow such professionals medical staff membership (absent state law to the contrary), although they could have clinical duties and responsibilities if permitted to do so by state law and the organization's medical staff bylaws. The new standard is permissive: if the medical staff determines that membership is appropriate, it is acceptable to JCAHO. The process of review and delineation of privileges is the same for all those who have independent clinical access to patients. Therefore, IAHPs undergo a similar credentialing process to determine the extent and scope of clinical privileges. As with physicians and dentists, renewal of privileges depends on continued and demonstrated competence in clinical performance.

The process of verifying a candidate's credentials begins when a clinician applies for medical staff membership and privileges. The process reviews all aspects of a candidate's education and training, licensure, and preparation. Controlling what a physician does is more difficult when procedures or activities are added to a set of privileges (i.e., when an orthopedic surgeon undertakes a hip replacement for the first time, when a neurosurgeon attempts an embolization of an arteriovenous shunt, when a cardiologist performs a catheterization using new techniques or equipment).

GUARANTEEING THE PATIENT'S SAFETY

Other issues that go beyond reviewing and approving the clinician's competence include: determining the presence of adequate support staff and equipment, evaluating the patient's clinical appropriateness for the procedure, and noting any deterioration in a clinician's capacity. Sometimes the problem is apparent only retrospectively. Ideally, the quality assurance process reviews the caregiver concurrently, if not prospectively.

Operating Beyond His Skill?

Jim Hudson picked up the form that had been delivered by the OR scheduling clerk and began to review the procedures scheduled for 2 days hence. Hudson's job is to ensure that there are adequate surgical packs, equipment, time, and personnel to meet the demands of surgery. Hudson immediately noticed a procedure that had never been on the schedule before. Looking at the column that indicated whether there would be need for

unusual equipment, Hudson saw a note that the attending surgeon would provide any special items. This puzzled him because it was the responsibility of the OR supervisor or the purchasing department to provide everything needed for a surgical
procedure. Hudson called the chief of surgery, to whom OR
staff reported clinically. He was unavailable, but his secretary
promised he would return the call.

When the chief of surgery called, he was noncommittal.
"If the procedure is scheduled," he said "it's probably okay for it
to be done." There was a clear implication that the surgeon
wouldn't perform a procedure with inadequate preparation.

Hudson wasn't sure what to do. As a nonphysician, any
further action by him would certainly be seen as meddling.
Nonetheless, it seemed necessary, perhaps even crucial.

This case focuses on a quality-assurance problem. Similar situations are
faced regularly by clinicians. Recent changes will make future monitoring and
review even more complex and problematic. Hudson must do more than ponder
the problem. Hudson should query the attending surgeon, and if that doesn't
produce satisfactory information, the problem should be taken higher up the
administrative hierarchy. Additional information may clear up the questions; it
may also cause the procedure to be cancelled.

As is true in all organizations and bureaucracies, health services professionals have a range of goals, objectives, and interests. A primary focus of their
lives is their work in the organization. It must be recognized, however, that
there is a limited congruence between personal goals and objectives and their
relationship with the organization. As noted in Chapter 3, employees must feel
that they and the organization have the same commitment to serving the patient.
This attitude must be reflected in action, not just the written organizational philosophy and policies.

If employees and medical staff perceive that the organization places greater
value on performance other than that reflecting ethical interaction with patients
(e.g., increasing hospital revenues), the principles of respect for persons, beneficence, and nonmaleficence will be in jeopardy. Since the organization acts
only through its staff, this lapse is serious. If staff fear that intervening on the
patient's behalf when necessary jeopardizes their relationship with the organization, they will be discouraged from acting as they should.

The "Uncooperative" RN

Sally Hansen, a registered nurse with 10 years experience,
regularly works nights. During rounds, she noted that a urinary
catheter had been ordered for a postsurgical patient with acute
urinary retention. Following established procedure, she paged
the resident on duty. A first-year resident appeared and told her
he would insert the catheter. Hansen accompanied him to the

bedside and observed him remove the catheter from its package. He looked at the package, apparently for instructions, but found none. The resident began to insert the catheter into the patient's penis, but faltered. It was apparent that he did not know what he was doing, and that the patient was experiencing great pain.

The resident turned and asked for assistance, but Hansen refused, saying that inserting a catheter was the job of a properly trained resident. "You really shouldn't attempt something you don't know how to do," she said. She also reminded the resident of hospital policy that prohibits a female nurse from performing certain intimate procedures on male patients. The resident yelled at the nurse and stalked off. Hansen called the chief resident, who catheterized the patient himself. He offered no explanation when Hansen described the incident with the inexperienced resident.

The next day, Hansen was awakened at home by a call from the vice president for nursing. She told Hansen that the inexperienced resident had filed a formal statement accusing her of insubordination. The resident was adamant about pressing the issue with nursing administration and the chief of his service. The vice president for nursing wasn't sure what the outcome would be.

What was Hansen's proper role in this matter? Where did her duties lie? Clearly, her duties lay with the patient and she acted properly. Even if she had known how to perform the procedure, she was constrained by hospital policy from performing it. By stopping the resident from continuing the procedure, she protected the patient from pain and potential injury. If Hansen is reprimanded by nursing administration, her willingness to intervene on a patient's behalf in the future will be reduced. Yet appropriate intervention by all staff is just what the hospital should be encouraging in order to gain the highest quality of care and to protect the patient.

This case brings out several issues. One is the traditional subservient role of nurses, probably due at least partly to sexism. Poor relations between doctors and nurses are not only a function of sexism, however. Anecdotal evidence suggests that the problem exists even where sexism is not a factor (i.e., male doctors and male nurses, female doctors and female nurses). Second, a resident is attempting a procedure that is beyond his competence. He should have had the good sense to get help on his own initiative. Third, there is an apparent lack of clarity as to the limits of residents' clinical activities. In this regard, the procedures and safeguards in the medical education program at the hospital may need review. Reinforcing Hansen's action, and in fact requiring it, is the American Nurses Association's Code for Nurses, which directs the nurse to act "to safeguard the client and the public when health care and safety are affected by the incompetent, unethical, or illegal practice of any person."[17] Implicit in this statement is accountability for one's actions as a nurse—an ethic—not merely accountability through the organizational hierarchy.

To assist personnel in cases such as these, the organization must make an unequivocal commitment that encourages staff to intervene when the patient is at risk. This policy should be communicated and enforced. Taking action in such cases may give rise to charges that caregivers are spying on one another. This charge is unfounded. Spying suggests a negative process—one that has no place in health services delivery. The focus here is on an organizationwide effort to protect and cure the patient. If caregivers are able to minimize their ego involvement in the care process and keep their eyes on these goals, this problem will be insignificant.

QUALITY ASSURANCE AND RISK MANAGEMENT

To obtain routine information on quality of services, health services organizations establish systems to review the content of clinical and administrative activities. Table 4 shows examples of quality measures. The parallels between the two types of activities are apparent. It should be stressed, however, that these are primarily objective functions and measures. The judgments and conclu-

Table 4. Some measures of hospital quality

Feature	Measures of patient care quality	Measures of administrative quality

Structure	Accreditation
	Medical staff qualifications
	Professional staff qualifications
	Professional staff training
	Special care unit availability/
	  utilization
		Accreditation
		Administrative staff qualifications
		Use of employee development
		  programs
		Personnel per occupied bed
		Services provided

Process	Medical staff audit Average length of stay Autopsy rate Community involvement	Use of management studies Occupancy rate Management planning activities Community involvement
Outcome	Patient outcome Surgical procedures assessment Adjusted death rate Hospital-acquired infections: reported/treated Malpractice suits	Cost per unit of output Man-hours per patient-day Financial stability

Attitude	Expert evaluation of patient care
	Patient satisfaction
	  (dissatisfaction)
		Expert evaluation of
		  administrative performance
		Employee satisfaction
		  (dissatisfaction)

Adapted from Grimes, R., and Moseley, Sik, "An Approach to an Index of Hospital Performance," *Health Services Research, 2* (Fall 1976): 289.

sions of those reviewing the data are also required. It is these conclusions that trigger action.

Consistent with the manager's duty to make patient well-being primary is the need to discourage or actively oppose establishing or continuing any service that exposes patients to unnecessary risk, whatever its source. One source of risk may be too low a volume of procedures. Early studies suggested that successful cardiac surgery was positively correlated with the number of procedures performed (i.e., hospitals performing fewer procedures of a particular type had worse results than hospitals performing more procedures). One factor that may have explained some of this difference—the acuity of illness of the patients being treated—received little attention, however. It may be that cardiac surgery programs that were willing to accept higher risk patients were those that performed fewer procedures. Absent that explanation, however, these studies recommended that low-volume/high-risk programs be closed. Later studies sustained these recommendations.

It has been suggested that the prospective payment system (diagnosis-related groups, or DRGs) will eliminate lower-volume higher-risk programs because these are also likely to have higher costs. This reasoning may be incorrect. It is possible for an unsuccessful program to be less expensive than a successful one. Therefore, less successful clinical programs might do well financially under DRGs, depending on other variables. If eliminating high-risk programs is justified, it must be done directly.

A major study of 266,944 patients sponsored by the National Center for Health Services Research (part of the Department of Health and Human Services) and reported in 1984 found that hospitals performing surgical procedures infreqently had a substantially higher death rate for patients than those with high volumes of the same operations. The study found that patients in nine surgical specialties had a 13% greater chance of dying if their operations were done in hospitals that performed relatively few operations. That study also found that patients in low-volume surgery hospitals tended to be hospitalized longer than those in high-volume institutions. In attempting to explain the findings, one of the authors noted:

> Individual staff members may become more highly qualified because of their increased experience in dealing with patients; organizational routines are more likely to be devised, and their regular use may enhance the performance of all participants; and specialized facilities and equipment may be more likely to be on hand.[18]

Similar results about the value of regionalizing in an effort to concentrate certain types of procedures, thus increasing volume, were obtained in other studies.[19] A study reported in 1989 confirmed the findings of the earlier studies, although it looked at physician volume rather than hospital volume.[20] Findings such as these have important implications for managers who either have a low-volume service or are considering undertaking one that is likely to remain a low-volume service.

Higher-Risk Procedures

Community Hospital was established in 1907 with a grant from a wealthy local industrialist. It has a long history of involvement in teaching activities, and provides education for nurses and physicians. Its surgical residency program is outstanding, and there are always many more applicants than openings. A keystone of the program has been thoracic surgery, in particular cardiac surgery. Two years ago, the cardiac surgery program was set back substantially as a result of the death of the chief of cardiac surgery and the departure of a member of the team. Referrals declined markedly and the volume of open-heart procedures dropped to five per month.

The quality assurance department performs special studies for various services in the hospital. Recently, it reviewed mortality data from the cardiac surgery program. The study found that mortality rates were more than double those reported in the literature. The director of quality assurance expressed concern as she discussed the report with the CEO. She noted that the literature reported an inverse relationship between mortality rates and the number of procedures performed. It seemed that technical competence could be gained only by performing a high volume of procedures.

Soon after, the CEO saw the medical director at lunch. During their conversation, the CEO asked whether he had any reason to believe that the cardiac surgery program was of lower quality than it had been in the past. The medical director replied, "As far as I know, things are fine." When he inquired as to the reason for the concern, the CEO replied that the frequency of performing cardiac procedures had declined, and the literature suggested that this had implications for the quality of care. In fact, the hospital's own quality assurance review had confirmed this. The medical director said he would look into it. The discussion moved to other matters.

The problem for Community Hospital and its patients is apparent to the CEO. It poses an ethical problem because patients undergoing cardiac surgery there are at higher risk than they would be elsewhere, thus violating the principle of nonmaleficence. The CEO may not ignore what is happening; to do so is inconsistent with the manager's role as a moral agent, as well as that of a professional with an independent duty to protect patients. What is the next step? Discontinuing the program immediately may be politically and economically impossible. But steps must be taken now to gain the support of the medical staff and to apprise the governing body of the problem. Whether or not the medical staff lends its support, the CEO must urge the governing body to suspend the program.

What happens if working within the organization proves fruitless because no one will listen? What if the problem is acknowledged, but those in power will not act? This situation causes a major test of the manager's ethic because it poses a true ethical dilemma. The manager is confronted with conflicting moral duties. On the one hand, information about the cardiac surgery program is confidential, and the manager has a duty of loyalty to the organization. On the other hand, organization inaction is putting patients at special risk. Weighing these conflicting duties should lead the manager to conclude that the higher duty is that of protecting patients. This means the manager must press and pursue— even to the point of releasing information outside the organization if corrective action is not taken. Going public with such damaging information (whistle-blowing) is a last resort. It is an act of great moral courage that requires a superior sense of conviction. Such an act will make the manager a pariah in the organization, someone who may be terminated for what is certain to be considered an act of betrayal.

The CEO might consider two other options that are more pragmatic, but ethically less desirable. One is to ignore the short-term implications of the decline in quality of care, and find and implement ways to build on program strengths, thereby increasing volume and quality. Another is to separate the types of procedures done into those significantly more and significantly less risky and to concentrate on performing those with less risk. Both approaches put patients at greater risk. This seems unconscionable in terms of the principles of beneficience and nonmaleficence, however. Absent an emergency or triage situation, one cannot justify the harm to some (patients) because of benefit to others (the surgeons and residents, and hospital income and reputation). Using patients as a means to an end is morally wrong.

RELATIONS WITH THE COMMUNITY

The health services organization is usually considered quasipublic, regardless of ownership. It has a service orientation and an ethical obligation to meet community health needs. This relationship necessitates building and retaining community confidence, and it means taking steps to act in the interests of persons in the community who are, as yet, only potential patients. If potential patients risk acquiring an infection or are in danger because the facility has physical plant or life safety code deficiencies, the organization has special obligations to them.

Protecting the Community

University Hospital has a unique role. It is a tertiary referral hospital for the region, and a major source of service to the community. In 1977, it experienced an outbreak of Legionella

(Legionnaires' disease). A number of patients contracted the disease; several died.

Legionnella is a bacterial infection of the respiratory tract and lungs that may result in death if not diagnosed and treated early. It is especially dangerous for elderly people and people with medical problems that weaken their general resistance. A factor requiring even greater caution on the part of hospital management is that at the time of the outbreaks, the process for identifying the organism in the laboratory took several days. Thus, patients were at greater risk until a confirmatory diagnosis was obtained.

Epidemiological studies showed a relationship between air conditioning cooling towers and the fine mist they give off, and spread of the disease through the aerosol. Workmen exposed directly to the aerosol have contracted severe cases of Legionnella. Chlorinating the water in the cooling towers eliminates the organism. Although a cooling tower was suspected in the 1977 outbreak at University Hospital, the relationship was never confirmed. The infection control committee of the hospital did not develop any standing orders or policies after the first outbreak.

In May, 1982, there was evidence of another outbreak of Legionnella. The cooling tower water was immediately chlorinated and the number of new cases dropped dramatically. However, an undetected failure in the chlorination system brought a second outbreak in early June.

When the first cases were detected in May, 1982, the administrator was notified. He met with various staff members, including physicians on the attending staff. It was decided that information about the outbreak should be kept from the community, lest there be a panic and sudden drop in census, as well as loss of public confidence. A confidential letter was sent to staff physicians advising them of the problem and asking that they keep in mind the potential for infection when making admissions decisions. However, admissions were not limited to emergencies, and there was no prospective review of elective admissions to determine whether patients at risk for pulmonary infections such as Legionnella should be sent elsewhere. Nor was there any review of indications for, and necessity of, admission. The medical staff developed a protocol stating that unexplained, acute-onset pneumonias were to be treated immediately with a very potent antibiotic known to be effective against Legionnella. However, no provision was made for effective review to determine that the protocol was actually followed.

The administrator at University Hospital faced several problems, all with ethical dimensions: 1) the medical staff wanted to continue admitting patients,

2) the community could lose confidence in the hospital if it learned that there was an epidemic of a potentially deadly disease, 3) the administrator and management staff could lose face or even their jobs should the infection become common knowledge, and 4) there was a potential for significant legal liability.

This management problem is difficult but by no means impossible to solve. Similar situations arise in nursing facilities (NFs) or intermediate care facilities (ICFs) that are threatened with closure because their physical plants violate fire safety requirements, and in hospitals in which outbreaks of meningitis or salmonella occur in the nursery. How does the organization protect current, as well as potential, patients in such situations? More importantly, what is the manager's role?

One feature that distinguishes the Legionnella outbreak from other similar cases is the difference in duty owed to potential versus actual patients. The law recognizes a difference. Generally, absent a special relationship with potential patients, one has no duty to act on their behalf. In this case, however, there would be a duty to warn elective admissions who are at risk from Legionnella.

The legal distinction is useful in an ethical analysis as well. The duty to assist actual patients is more immediate and more compelling than the duty toward potential patients. Even potential patients should not be put at risk, however, unless their medical condition puts them at greater risk outside the hospital than inside it. Inpatients who might benefit from a continued stay but who are at greater risk by remaining in the hospital should be discharged. It is incumbent on the managerial and clinical staff to make those involved in care understand the obligation to protect the patient.

The argument that the administrator has a duty to protect the reputation of the organization in the community has merit because persons needing hospitalization should have no fear about getting it and because of the significant psychological component in health care. Furthermore, persons may be at greater risk by not obtaining treatment for their medical problems than they are from Legionnella. Yet they may defer care because they are frightened or lack confidence in the facility.

At admission, potential risk becomes actual risk. Emergency admissions do not pose an ethical problem assuming there is no alternative source of care and the risk of no care is greater than that of contracting Legionnella.

Elective admissions are quite different. At the very least, the organization, led and prompted by its managers, should have developed and applied policies and procedures separating high-risk from low-risk elective admissions and made special provisions either to send the former group elsewhere or to take special efforts to protect them. Ethically, it could not rely on the discretion of the admitting physician. As with any quality-assurance activity, management has a responsibility to review decision making about care and to do so in a fashion consistent with the level of risk. Here, that means concurrent review.

The potential conflicts of interest are obvious. It is natural for managers to protect their positions and reputations. They do this out of loyalty to the organization, but also out of selfish interests. A typical response is to cover up. Concealment seems like an easy way to reduce the risk of personal and professional damage. Experience suggests, however, that not only from an ethical but also from a pragmatic standpoint, honesty is the best policy. Rumors are certain to be carried into the community by staff and patients, and the potential tarnish on the organization's reputation may be much longer lasting than if the community is informed that there is a problem and that steps are being taken to protect patients from infection. This tactic may raise questions about the cause of and responsibility for the problem, but the community will not mistrust the organization. Furthermore, in terms of guiding ethical principles, the organization is treating people in the community with respect and dignity by being truthful.

The health services organization loses community confidence when it no longer appears to have the community's best interests in mind. Here the conflict is between protecting the organization's financial integrity—an ethical obligation of the organization linked to its role of providing services to the community—and that of serving an individual patient.

How Can We Afford This?

A 63-year-old woman slipped into an irreversible coma after suffering two heart attacks. Three years later she was still a patient in an acute care hospital. Her aggregate unpaid bill totaled $750,000 after private insurance coverage lapsed. The insurer argued that the patient was receiving only custodial care, and it would therefore not pay for acute care. The patient could be transferred to another facility only if she were declared mentally incompetent. Hospital efforts to achieve this caused much adverse publicity in the community and subsequent court action. Ultimately, the hospital failed to achieve its goal of moving the woman out of the facility.

The organization and its managers faced an ethical dilemma—they had an ongoing relationship with a patient who no longer needed acute care. The principles of beneficience and nonmaleficence prevented them from abandoning the patient, but the uncompensated costs of her care increasingly conflicted with the hospital's obligation to maintain its financial integrity—the principle of justice in allocating resources. It seems trite to characterize the results in this case as a public relations failure, but the hospital might have gained community understanding had it been more forthright and communicative in describing the problem and the dilemma it faced as it sought to move the woman into a suitable alternative facility.

CONCLUSION

Nonphysician managers do not personally judge the quality of clinical activities. They are, however, responsible for providing clinical staff with the systems, procedures, and resources required to do an effective job. As suggested by the principles of beneficence and nonmaleficence, managers must have enough awareness of what is expected and how that expection is measured to determine that the goal of delivering quality health services has been met. Managers are remiss in their ethical (and legal) duties if they occupy themselves exclusively with nonclinical activities and claim that clinical matters lie outside their ken and range of responsibilities. Just as they rely on computer programmers or wage and salary experts for reports, advice, and counsel, so too, managers rely on technical expertise and assistance in judging patient care. The manager is accountable to the governing body for all activities, and this requires active involvement and effective partnerships between managers and clinicians.

This chapter identifies and discusses several generic ethical problems arising out of the duties owed by managers to patients and community. The duties are not always clear and may be further obscured by accompanying problems, such as bureaucratic inertia and medical staff relations. However, they become clear if managers focus on the primary reasons for the organization's existence—serving and protecting the patient and community.

NOTES

1. James S. Bowman, Frederick A. Elliston, and Paula Lockhart, eds., *Professional Dissent: An Annotated Bibliography and Research Guide,* vol. 2 (New York: Garland Publishing, 1984), 3.

2. Myron Glazer, "Ten Whistleblowers and How They Fared," *Hastings Center Report 13,* no. 6 (December 1983): 33–41.

3. Alan F. Westin, *Whistle Blowing! Loyalty and Dissent in the Corporation* (New York: McGraw-Hill, 1981).

4. Ibid., 139.

5. Ibid., 140.

6. Ibid.

7. Ibid., 144.

8. "Potential Whistle Blowers Fear Reprisal," *Washington Post,* January 18, 1985.

9. Bowman, Elliston, and Lockhart, *Professional Dissent,* 4.

10. *O'Sullivan v. Mallon et al.,* 160 N.J. Super. 416, 390 A.2d 149 (1978).

11. *Pierce v. Ortho Pharmaceuticals,* 84 N.J. 58, 417 A.2d 505 (1980).

12. *O'Sullivan v. Mallon et al.*

13. *Commonwealth of Pennsylvania ex rel. Rafferty et al. v. Philadelphia Psychiatric Center,* 356 F. Supp. 500 (E.D. Pa. 1973).

14. Lawrence Blades, "Employment at Will vs. Individual Freedom: On Limiting the Abusive Exercise of Employer Power," *Columbia Law Review 67* (December 1967): 1407.

15. Westin, *Whistle Blowing,* 133–136.

16. Ibid., 142.

17. American Nurses Association, "Code for Nurses," 1976.

18. Spencer Rich, "Hospitals Doing More Operations Lose Fewer Patients," *Washington Post,* April 26, 1984.

19. Harold S. Luft, John P. Bunker, and Alain C. Enthoven, "Should Operations be Regionalized?" *New England Journal of Medicine 301,* no. 25 (December 1979): 1364–1369.

20. Edward L. Hannan, Joseph F. O'Donnell, Harold Kilburn, Jr., Harvey R. Bernard, and Altan Yazici, "Investigation of the Relationship Between Volume and Mortality for Surgical Procedures Performed in New York State Hospitals," *Journal of the American Medical Association 262,* no. 4 (July 1989): 503–510.

IV

∞

BIOMEDICAL ETHICAL ISSUES

THIS PART ADDRESSES THE BIOMEDICAL ETHICAL issues most often confronted by health services organizations and their managers. They include consent, death and dying, experimentation, and abortion. A myriad of other biomedical ethical issues include: genetic engineering, screening, and counseling; psychosurgery and behavior control; the right to health care; infanticide and the rights of the fetus; truth telling in medicine; concepts of personhood; rights and responsibilities of patients; implants and transplants; and mental illness and involuntary commitment. Several of these issues were addressed tangentially in Part III in terms of their effect on the manager. Space limitations prevent considering them further.

The thorny issue of consent is addressed in Chapter 9. It affects managers in all types of health services organizations. The legal system has defined the acceptable relationship between provider and patient, but managers should consider this only a starting point—one built upon by their efforts as moral agents.

Chapter 10 addresses the biomedical ethical issues surrounding death and dying. Significant changes during the past 2 decades, many resulting from the effects of technology, have raised many new issues here. Chapter 10 is divided into defining death; applying life-sustaining treatment (using the example of infants with impairments); withdrawing treatment; and the ethical aspects of intervening in the terminal stages of life. Few health services organizations are unaffected by all of these aspects of death and dying and, like consent, these issues have major implications for managers.

Chapter 11 addresses the issues of experimentation and abortion. They have common ground in fetal research. In the main, however, they are distinct issues with distinct ethical implications for managers. Managers should not consider research an issue limited to the university medical center. Innovative therapy is an aspect of research and can affect any organization. Abortion is an issue that has been addressed by virtually every acute care organization. Those with an ill-defined philosophy have had, and will continue to have, problems over the ethical aspects of abortion.

9

∞

CONSENT

Consent is an ethical imperative of great importance to managers and clinicians. In its study of consent, the President's Commission found that patients generally want to be more involved in the decision-making process. This finding suggests both a problem and a goal for health services providers.

The concept of consent evolved to protect persons from nonconsensual touching. Although the ethical and legal aspects of consent overlap greatly, the law of consent is only a minimum requirement. In terms of ethics, consent is expanded and is based on the principle of respect for persons—specifically, autonomy, which reflects a view of the equality and dignity of human beings. To a lesser extent the concept of consent reflects the special relationship of trust and confidence between physician and patient, and between organization and patient. It is supported by the principles of beneficence and nonmaleficence.

At law, a failure to obtain proper consent can result in a legal action for battery, an intentional tort. Beyond this, an action for negligence can be brought if the physician breaches the duty to communicate the information necessary for the patient to give consent that is informed.

Paternalism is based on the principle of beneficence and is the ethical value competing with autonomy in efforts to implement consent. Paternalism arises naturally from the relationship between physician and patient because psychologically, technically, and emotionally, the physician is in a position of superior knowledge, and may be expected to choose the best course of action for the patient. Historically, the paternalistic nature of physician–patient relations can be traced to the Hippocratic Oath. The sense of beneficence and paternalism continues to be the dominant, implicit theme in the practice of medicine (albeit implicitly). The Principles of Medical Ethics adopted by the American Medical Association (AMA) in 1980 suggest new directions for organized medicine, however—away from paternalism and toward autonomy and patient rights. The AMA Principles are reproduced in Appendix B.

Specialized codes, such as the Declaration of Helsinki, which guides biomedical research, also recognize the importance of consent. The emphasis on patients' rights or sovereignty in documents such as these are ideals toward which the organization should strive.

LEGAL CONSIDERATIONS

Consent must be voluntary, competent, and informed. These requirements do not apply in an emergency, when the law presumes that persons want to receive treatment. If, however, the person needing treatment is competent, or if someone authorized to speak for the person is present, consent must be obtained. When minors or people who are mentally incompetent are patients, and those who speak for them refuse to give consent, the organization is usually successful in persuading the state to authorize treatment.

Typically, even in a nonemergency, general consent for treatment is implied by the patient's presence and apparent desire to be treated. Noninvasive elective treatment of a routine nature requires only general consent. For invasive, surgical, or special procedures, or when the patient is part of an experiment, special consent is needed. Oral consent is as meaningful legally as written consent, but personnel turnover, faulty memories, and prudence make it imperative that consent be written. General and special consent forms are shown in Figures 8 and 9.

As noted, consent has three elements: voluntary, competent, and informed. To be *voluntary,* consent must be given without duress that significantly influences the decision. Whether duress is excessive depends on the facts. Using threats or force clearly constitutes duress. In some circumstances persons have diminished autonomy. The military or prison are examples. In the past, these settings were used for research involving human subjects. Recent publicity and subsequent public indignation have greatly reduced the amount of experimentation performed on persons in such settings, however.

Competent consent means that the patient knows the nature and consequences of the course of treatment under consideration. The law presumes minor children are incompetent. In addition, people whose mental illness or mental disability has caused them to be found legally incompetent are not permitted to make decisions regarding medical treatment or experimentation. Other people must make such decisions for them. Questions of mental competence become very complex, however, when patients are terminally ill, depressed, or suicidal.

Finally, consent must be *informed.* The law requires full disclosure of the nature of the patient's condition and the treatment proposed, the alternatives available, and the likely consequences and difficulties that might result from treatment or nontreatment. The majority of courts has held that patients should receive as much information as the reasonable physician would give under similar or identical circumstances. A minority of courts has established standards based on what the typical patient would want to know. A legal criterion used by a few courts—and one more oriented to patient sovereignty—is what that particular patient would have wanted to know.

When issues of family obligations arise in cases involving Jehovah's Witnesses, a religion that prohibits transfusions of whole blood, some courts order

The George Washington University/Medical Center

Authorization for Medical Care and Treatment
Authorization for Release of Medical Records to Third-Party Payers
Release of Responsibility for Personal Property/Valuables

1. I have come to George Washington University's Hospital for medical treatment. I ask the health care professionals at the Hospital to provide care and treatment for me that they feel is necessary. I consent to undergo routine tests and treatment as part of this care. I understand that I am free to ask a member of my health care team questions about any care, treatment or medicine I am to receive.

2. Because George Washington University's Hospital is a teaching hospital, I understand that my health care team will be made up of hospital personnel and medical students in addition to my attending physician and his/her assistants and designees. Hospital personnel include, but are not limited to, nurses, technicians, interns, residents, and fellows.

3. I understand that as part of my care and treatment, samples of my blood, urine, stool and tissues may be removed from me from time to time. I permit the University to use any leftover blood, urine, stool and tissues for research. (If I do not want the University to so use leftover portions, I may stop the University from doing so by writing "no" in the following block and writing my initials after it [   ].) If additional samples are needed for the research, I will be asked at that time.

4. I am aware that the practice of medicine is not an exact science and admit that no one has given me any promises or guarantees about the result of any care or treatment I am to receive or examinations I am to undergo.

5. I agree to the University's and/or my physician sending copies of my medical records (or information from my medical records) to my insurance provider(s) or other sources of payment, which may include my employer. I understand that this information will be sent when it is needed for payment of my medical bills. I release and forever discharge The George Washington University, its employees and agents and my attending physician from any liability resulting from the release of my medical records or information from them for payment purposes.

6. **Release of Responsibility for Personal Property/Valuables:** I understand that George Washington University is not responsible for any personal property or valuables that I keep with me while I am at the hospital, even if placed in a hospital provided locker. Personal property includes, but is not limited to, clothing, shoes and baggage. Valuables include, but are not limited to, money, credit cards, dentures, eyeglasses, hearing aids and jewelry. I understand, therefore, that I should send my valuables and as much of my property as possible home with my family/friends. I realize that I can request the University's Cashier's Office to store valuables I cannot send home.

7. I am currently a Tissue/Organ donor: ☐ YES   ☐ NO

EMERGENCY UNIT PATIENTS ONLY

8. I understand that it may be helpful for my personal physician to be involved in the care I receive while I am in The George Washington University Emergency Unit. I therefore allow an Emergency Unit physician to contact my personal physician, Dr. _____. (If I do not wish my physician to be contacted, I may stop the University from doing so by writing "no" in the following block and writing my initials after it. [   ].)

9. I agree to the University's sending copies of my Emergency Unit record to my personal physician named above. (If I do not wish the University to send a copy to my physician, I may stop the University from doing so by writing "no" in the following block and writing my initials after it. [   ].)

AFFIRMATION

I have read this form and understand it. All of my questions about what it says have been answered. I am signing it of my own free will. I understand that by signing it, I am agreeing to it.

_____   _____
Signature of patient (or parent, legal guardian or   Date/Time
next-of-kin. Please indicate which.)

_____   _____
Witness to affirmation and signature   Date/Time

Figure 8.   A general consent form. (From The George Washington University Medical Center, Washington, DC. Reprinted with permission.)

treatment. On two occasions, Maryland Circuit Court Judge John J. McAuliffe ordered transfusions for patients in suburban Washington, D.C. hospitals. In both cases, the patients were parents with significant family responsibilities. One patient had five children, who the judge ruled would be emotionally and psychologically deprived if their mother died; the other patient was the sole support of a wife and 2-year-old son.[1] However, in a similar case, a judge in the

I, Haskell Karp, request and authorize Dr. Denton A. Cooley and such other surgeons as he may designate to perform upon me, in St. Luke's Episcopal Hospital of Houston, Texas, cardiac surgery for advanced cardiac decompensation and myocardial insufficiency as a result of numerous coronary occlusions. The risk of this surgery has been explained to me. In the event cardiac function cannot be restored by excision of destroyed heart muscle and plastic reconstruction of the ventricle and death seems imminent, I authorize Dr. Cooley and his staff to remove my diseased heart and insert a mechanical cardiac substitute. I understand that this mechanical device will not be permanent and ultimately will require a replacement by a heart transplant. I realize that this device has been tested in the laboratory but has not been used to sustain a human being and that no assurance of success can be made. I expect the surgeons to exercise every effort to preserve my life through any of these means. No assurance has been made by anyone as to the results that may be obtained.

I understand that the operating surgeon will be occupied solely with the surgery and that the administration of the anesthetic(s) is an independent function. I hereby request and authorize Dr. Arthur S. Keats, or others he may designate, to administer such anesthetics as he or they may deem advisable.

I hereby consent to the photographing of the operation to be performed, including appropriate portions of my body, for medical, scientific, and educational purposes.

_____   _____
Signature   Date

Figure 9. A special consent form (From *Karp v. Cooley*, 349 F. Supp. 827 [S.D. Texas 1972]; aff'd, 493 F 2d 408 [5th Cir. 1974], cert. denied, 419 U.S. 845 [1974].)

same geographic area but a different jurisdiction permitted a patient to refuse a blood transfusion even though his life was at stake. The affected family in that case had a good economic situation and a strong family network to support the wife and her children. Despite the dire predictions, the patient recovered.[2] These cases show that judges have considered more than a liberty right such as autonomy when more important societal interests are present.

An ethic that emphasizes autonomy and the respect owed individuals has a significant effect on how patients are treated in health services organizations. This ethic requires that the patient be actively involved in the process of care. The President's Commission stated that patient sovereignty, with complete participation in the process, is desirable, although not a readily achievable goal.[3] The goal of participation cannot be achieved and the principle of respect for persons realized, however, in the absence of truthfulness and the organization's consistent effort to perfect the participation (autonomy) of patients. Participation means that the patient may not agree with caregivers' recommendations and assessments. Some clinicians and some organizations find this threatening.

Some patients do not wish to participate in decision making. Explicitly or implicitly, they want to remain ignorant about their medical problems and be excluded from decision processes. They prefer a paternalistic relationship, and they choose to delegate decision making and allow those caring for them to do what they think best. This is not the relationship between patient and caregivers envisoned by the President's Commission, but patients' autonomy is also violated if they are forced to participate. Caregivers and managers should consider a decision not to participate an acceptable choice, and work to make it a reality.

There is in the law a concept known as *therapeutic privilege*. It permits physicians to withhold information from patients when they consider doing so to be in the patients' best interests. States recognize therapeutic privilege in a variety of ways; a general rule is difficult to state. They include criteria that reference danger to the patient's physical or mental health if there is full disclosure, as well as criteria that are concerned with the patient's best interests.[4] This paternalistic view of the patient arises from the principles of beneficence and nonmaleficence. The therapeutic privilege exception is pragmatic. It permits physicians a broader range of actions. It is desirable that physicians have the latitude to make such judgments, especially if the alternative is greater harm to the patient. Here, the principle of beneficence is deemed more important and takes precedence.

ETHICAL CONSIDERATIONS

This discussion of the ethics of consent begins with the premise that the ethical standard must be significantly higher than the legal standard. This ethical standard is drawn from the principles of respect for persons (autonomy) and nonmaleficence, which are in turn based on Kantian deontology, natural law, and rule utilitarianism.

In determining whether consent is voluntary, nuances of duress and inducement are important. Here, ethical considerations and duties go far beyond the minimum standard established by the law. Can patients suffering from an often fatal disease make medical decisions voluntarily? Can patients make a decision free of duress if they fear loss of their physicians' friendship and loyalty because they prefer an option their physician opposes? Clinical personnel speak about "bad" patients—patients who are uncooperative. Although not intentionally harmed or mistreated, such patients may not receive the same level of attention as "good," or pliable, patients. Patients sense this, and it affects their volition. In addition, patients are heavily influenced by family and friends, and may make decisions because of them. Similarly, family members ask health care providers to act in ways that may not be wanted by the incapacitated patient, or that, under the principle of beneficence, are not in the patient's interests.

Given these considerations, is consent ever voluntary? It has been argued that patients' personal freedom to accept or reject medical treatment has been reduced to the point that it exists only as a right to veto unwanted procedures.[5] The complex relationships in medical care preclude simple answers and easy determinations as to the voluntariness of consent. It is critical, however, that the organization's managerial and clinical staff understand this and make every effort to further patient autonomy.

Some groups present special problems in terms of determining the voluntariness of consent. For example, persons with diminished autonomy, such as soldiers or prisoners, sometimes participate in nontherapeutic experimentation (experimentation that holds no benefit for the subject). Since their status limits autonomy, is their consent truly voluntary? Voluntariness may also be reduced through inducements of such magnitude that caution and prudence are cast aside. For example, large amounts of money may be offered for participation in a potentially dangerous experiment, or a low level of compensation may be offered to people whose economic position is such that even modest rewards constitute undue inducement. Students are unique in this regard and may fit more than one category. They are often economically disadvantaged. In addition, some academic courses encourage them to participate in experiments by exempting them from other, seemingly more onerous requirements, such as examinations. There is also implicit, or sometimes explicit, coercion by faculty members who control the students' academic (and sometimes economic) destiny, and who unethically use this position to coerce consent.

Ethical considerations regarding competence for consent are simpler than those surrounding the voluntariness of consent. Competence is assumed in adults. Medical personnel can usually determine when a patient's mental capacity is questionable, and obtain an expert opinion. Absent such evidence, there should be an explicit presumption in the organization that patients can exercise their autonomy and make their own decisions. It is incumbent on managers to assist in this process through education and support from systems and procedures.

The third element of consent is that it be informed. Some commentators inaccurately refer to the concept of "informed consent" as though being informed were the only aspect of consent. Because it is the most complex element, whether the patient was adequately informed receives the most attention. Several states have statutes to aid patients in obtaining information for an informed decision. The Virginia law was prompted by reports that physicians were performing radical mastectomies when removal of the malignant tumor would suffice, and it was claimed that women were not given enough information to make an intelligent choice. When introduced, the proposal raised questions among a number of groups, including the American Cancer Society, which said the emphasis should be on improved education about the disease and alternative methods of treatment, rather than a legislative enactment.[6]

Wait a Little Longer, We'll Do it Then

The emergency department at County Hospital experienced a typical caseload: many true emergencies, and a lot of sniffles and other nonemergencies. It had a contract with an emergency medicine specialty group, but all the administrative activities, including systems, procedures, and personnel, were managed by the hospital. The process for obtaining consent was typical. Unconscious emergency patients were treated as indicated. Patients able to communicate signed a consent authorizing treatment. Parents and next of kin were involved as needed and as available.

Early one afternoon, a conscious, middle-aged male was brought in. He had been in a car accident and was diagnosed as having internal injuries requiring immediate exploratory surgery. When asked to sign the consent form, he refused on the grounds that he was a Christian Scientist and receiving medical treatment violated his religious beliefs. He asked for a Christian Science reader.

The physician director of the emergency department had been paged. After hearing the facts about the patient, the director was sure she could obtain his consent for surgery. She briefly discussed the alternatives with the patient. He clearly understood that without surgery, death would be almost certain. He persisted in refusing to consent, and repeatedly asked for a reader. When the director left the treatment room, she was very agitated and her mouth and chin shook in anger. She said, "This man is throwing his life away, all in the name of some religion that denies scientific medicine to its adherents. I can't believe he's doing it!" She turned to the nurse and said in a whisper, "Let me know when he's unconscious and we'll save his life, despite his silly ideas."

The physician plans to do to a patient when he is unconscious what he forbade her to do when he was conscious. This deception rides roughshod over the patient's clearly expressed wishes. The patient is competent, he has been informed, and his refusal is voluntary. In addition to violating the principle of respect for persons (autonomy), the physician is ignoring the AMA's Principles of Medical Ethics. Such methods are unconscionable.

The organizational philosophy should address such issues prospectively. The results could reflect the same approach used in the case of Baby Boy Doe, in Chapter 1. There, it was suggested that the organization might choose to intervene by petitioning a court to order life-saving surgery. This gives less weight to the principle of respect for persons (autonomy) and more to the principle of beneficence, and its corollary, utility. The result for the Christian Scientist could be a decision that he and society benefit if he is kept alive. Since the patient is saved with relative ease, the principle of nonmaleficence also supports a decision to act, even though acting is contrary to the patient's wishes. The patient might have a family to whom he has obligations. Requiring treatment in such cases is paternalistic and significantly limits individual autonomy.

Because of competing ethical principles, cases such as these pose ethical dilemmas for the organization and its managers.

ROLE OF THE ORGANIZATION

What is the organization's role? Patients should give informed, voluntary, and competent consent before treatment. This is a simple ethical principle. As is often the case, however, difficulties arise in the application of this principle, and it is here that the criteria may be more often violated than met. Recently, organizations have given greater attention to consent. This emphasis usually reflects fear of legal problems, rather than the desire to do what is ethically correct. In the past, organizations were less concerned about consent, because they adopted and amplified the paternalistic view of the patient historically found in medicine.

At the very least, policies and procedures consistent with the organizational philosophy must be established for obtaining consent, and their application must be systematically monitored. If the philosophy emphasizes patients' rights, actions and efforts to guarantee those rights will be encouraged, and actions and efforts to contravene them will be restricted. There are specific means for allowing patients to assert their rights, but they are costly and can become adversarial. One way is to provide a patient representative for each patient. Another is to establish an office of ombudsman to review problems.

Often, the circumstances of consent are complicated because of the many parties involved—providers, patient, and family.

When is Consent Consent?

Henry Franklin was admitted to University Hospital through the emergency department. He was diagnosed by one of the attending staff as having mild cardiac failure. Because of his age (78) and other complicating medical problems, there was a dispute as to the proper course of treatment. The cardiologist who consulted on the case recommended that Franklin be treated medically and given the best quality of life possible. The cardiologist estimated his remaining life at 6 months.

The cardiac surgeons had a different view of suitable treatment. They recommended replacing the aortic and mitral valves and estimated this would provide at least 2 years of useful life. When the options were described to Franklin, he was told there was a 50-50 probability he could survive the surgery. He decided he would work with the cardiologist to have the best possible quality of life.

After hearing his decision, the surgeons intervened directly with Franklin's family. The family agreed with the surgeons and put great pressure on Franklin. He finally agreed to the procedure. Franklin did not withstand the surgery and died in the operating room.

However informed or competent, Franklin's final decision was made under great stress. The circumstances under which consent was given were almost coercive. In situations such as this, family and physicians seem to be acting in a patient's best interests, but sometimes both relatives and caregivers are driven by conflicting motives.

The basic problem for managers is to ensure patient autonomy. Patients may choose a course of action that is not their first choice, nor even in their own best interests as they view them, because they defer to the wishes of family, friends, or employers. They may also fear abandonment or the anger of care-givers if they choose to do something other than what the caregivers think is wanted of them. An added complexity is that patients themselves are often uncertain about what to do—they vacillate between wanting and not wanting aggressive treatment. Preserving patient autonomy in these circumstances is difficult, but must be attempted nonetheless.

For Franklin, the surgeons played an important role. They may have allowed bravado to cloud good judgment, especially given the probability of success. Franklin's relatives were important, too, and the health services organization interferes at its peril in situations that reflect usual family dynamics, even though it has a duty to protect the patient and further his interests.

What is the role of the organization in determining that patients have consented in a way that meets ethical criteria? Obvious coercion is likely to be noticed by the staff. A patient representative program may help minimize duress. Complicating efforts to ensure that consent meets the criteria is that the private attending physician has an independent ethical duty to inform patients about the nature of the medical procedure. The attending physician is also primary in determining that the patient is competent to give consent, and does so voluntarily. Some health services organizations make an independent determination that the criteria of consent have been met. Others ask only that patients sign an authorization verifying that they have been informed about the procedure by the physician and permitting the hospital to participate in rendering the care to which the physician and patient have agreed. Unless the organization is certain that patients have been adequately informed about the procedure, the ethically preferred course is to inform them independently. The manager must fulfill the organization's positive ethical duty to monitor consent processes. It is critical to establish a process, including forms and procedures, to assist and guide staff. In addition, physician and nonphysician staff will benefit from education about the ethical (and legal) dimensions of consent.

The case of Henry Franklin is distinguishable from that of the Christian Scientist. Franklin had more time to consider his decision, which was undoubtedly influenced by his age. The other patient was middle aged, with many productive and enjoyable years ahead of him. Beyond these apparent differences, however, the cases raise questions about patient autonomy and its relationship to the principles of beneficence and nonmaleficence. The weight given these principles in the organizational philosophy determines the outcome.

In terms of consent, managers of nursing facilities (NFs) face ethical issues very similar to those faced by their counterparts in acute care hospitals. In NFs, decision making is frequently complicated by other factors, such as competence or abandonment of patients, however. Thus, there is need for special attention to the process.

I Mean to Be Independent

Oliver Harris had been a resident at Five Oaks Nursing Home for almost 5 years. When he first sought admission, Harris had been evaluated and found only marginally in need of the skilled care provided at Five Oaks. He was a private pay patient, however, and management had decided to admit him. For over 3 years, his health had been such that he needed only the minimum of skilled nursing. In his 5th year, he showed evidence of dementia. Medical evaluation showed that he had had several minor strokes. Harris was very active physically, and had always done a great deal of walking in the facility. He liked to visit other patients as he went around the facility. His declining medical condition had resulted in several falls, however, which had caused some cuts and bruises, but, as yet, no broken bones.

Harris was discussed at a staff conference. It was the consensus that he should be restrained so that he could not ambulate independently, but this was possible under the new OBRA guidelines only if Harris's physician was willing to order restraints. It was doubtful that the physician would agree with the staff recommendation. The staff believed that if he continued to walk on his own it was only a matter of time before he fell and broke a bone. The decision was discussed with Harris, but he was adamant that he not be restrained. His daughter was called and she agreed with the staff. The staff believe, too, that even if restraints were ordered by the physicians, Harris would fight them in every way he could.

The staff and management face a dilemma. How are they to meet their duty of nonmaleficence to Harris while at the same time meeting their obligation to maximize his autonomy under the principle of respect for persons? Harris is competent to make a decision regarding restraints. It is clear, too, that he is risking his continued well-being. If, for example, he falls, breaks a bone, and is hospitalized, his general health is likely to deteriorate rapidly. The staff do not seem to be very creative in finding a way to allow him to ambulate safely. Such possibilities should be explored first. Alternatively, various options should be tried for short periods. If all efforts fail, however, and Harris cannot be persuaded to accept restraints, nothing should be done to interfere with his freedom to ambulate in the facility.

MEDICAL EDUCATION

The case of Richard Weidner included in Chapter 8 involves problems of consent in the context of medical education. Weidner was admitted to the hospital for a cardiac catheterization following recurrent chest pain. His cardiologist told him she would perform the procedure, but it was actually done by a cardiology resident. The misrepresentation violated Weidner's right to autonomy and informed decision making, and angered him considerably.

Medical education is a major source of problems concerning consent, especially in terms of the information about who will perform a particular procedure. In January, 1978, a Medical Practice Task Force established by the New York State Assembly issued its report. The report's conclusions were not based on statistical evidence of harm to patients caused by residents performing surgery, but on interviews with chiefs of surgery, attending surgeons, residents, and anesthesiologists at 34 hospitals in New York state. It reported that:

- Private surgical patients in teaching hospitals are usually not operated on by the attending surgeon they retained, but by residents. Between 50% and 85% of the surgery in teaching hospitals is done by residents.
- Although most residents operated only under the close supervision of attending surgeons, some residents performed surgery without supervision, and some attending surgeons left the room while the operation was still in progress or before the incision was closed.
- Most patients are unaware of the degree to which residents participate in their surgery, and consent forms that name the attending surgeon and "such assistants as he shall select" do not give patients meaningful notice that a resident may do the actual cutting or suturing.[7]

The authors stressed there was no evidence that allowing residents to be major participants in surgery caused harm to patients. Other researchers are less certain in this regard, however. They suggest that harm to patients from care rendered by physicians in training may be much more common than generally known.[8] Whether or not harm is done is a utilitarian consideration. Kantians do not consider outcomes, but only determine whether actions meet the criterion of respect for persons. Misleading patients or lying to them violates this principle.

Recommendations to the legislature resulting from the report focused on providing the disclosure necessary for informed consent and having sufficient supervision to ensure patient safety. It was recommended that physicians be required to obtain the patient's consent for each person who participates in the surgery. It also recommended that vague phrases such as "such assistants as the surgeon may select" be deleted from consent forms. The recommendations encouraged adequate supervision by limiting the number of patients a surgeon could treat and the number of operating rooms that surgeons could reserve at one time.[9]

The AMA and American College of Surgeons (ACS) have addressed this question. Both believe that if a resident, rather than the surgeon retained by the patient, actually performs the surgery, the patient must be made aware of that fact, and consent to the substitution. "Current Opinions of the Judicial Council of the AMA" states:

> A surgeon who allows a substitute to operate on his patient without the patient's knowledge and consent is deceitful. The patient is entitled to choose his own physician and he should be permitted to acquiesce in or refuse to accept the substitution. . . .
>
> Under the normal and customary agreement with patients, and with reference to the usual form of consent to operation, the operating surgeon is obligated to perform the operation but may be assisted by residents or other surgeons. With the consent of the patient, it is not unethical for the operating surgeon to delegate the performance of certain aspects of the operation to his assistant provided this is done under his participatory supervision, i.e., he must scrub. If a resident or other physician is to perform the operation under nonparticipatory supervision, it is necessary to make a full disclosure of this fact to the patient, and this should be evidenced by an appropriate statement contained in the consent. Under these circumstances, it is the resident or other physician who becomes the operating surgeon.[10]

In its Statements on Principles, the ACS states:

> A surgeon may delegate part of the care of his patient to associates or residents under his direction, because modern surgery is often a team effort, but he must not delegate or evade his responsibility. It is proper for the responsible surgeon to delegate the performance of part of a given operation to his assistants, provided the surgeon is an active participant throughout the essential part of the operation. If a resident is to operate upon and take care of the patient, under the general supervision of an attending surgeon who will not participate actively, the patient should be so informed and consent thereto.
>
> It is unethical to mislead a patient as to the identity of the doctor who performs the surgery. . . .[11]

These statements are unequivocal. The patient must be told about the participation of a resident. Regrettably, the evidence suggests that these principles are regularly violated. Learning by doing is most apparent in training surgeons. It is also present, however, when residents in medicine are educated. Ethically, there is no difference between a surgical resident wielding a scalpel on an unsuspecting patient or a medical resident ordering that a patient be injected with a medication.

Inadequate attention is paid to consent. It is an area in which patient autonomy is often breached, and in which organizations through their managers must substantially improve performance. Medical education and patient consent are compatible. Most patients will cooperate when they have knowledge that physicians in training are to have a role in their care.[12] If patients are unwilling to permit residents to treat them to the point where they seek care elsewhere, this is their right. If this right is ignored, attention to patient rights and autonomy is lacking.

CONCLUSION

This chapter addresses ethical issues raised by consent. The health services organization and its managers should consider legal constraints as only a minimum standard. It is on the basis of ethical principles that the organization should build a strong relationship with the patient. This independent relationship is the basis for the autonomy and respect owed the patient.

Operationalizing the President's Commission's finding that patients desire to be more involved in the consent process will require managerial attention to consent processes. The task will not be easy. It requires overcoming a long history of medical paternalism. It means educating patients, as well as encouraging and assisting them to become involved.

A major problem is providing information about their treatment to patients hospitalized in teaching institutions. Managers will have an uphill struggle in convincing attending staff that fully informing patients will not lead to a diminution in clinical material for teaching programs. There is no evidence to suggest, however, that large numbers of patients will refuse to participate after they have been informed; there is every reason to believe that, overwhelmingly, patients will agree to resident involvement.

NOTES

1. Tom Vesey, "Judge Orders Transfusions for Mother Near Death," *Washington Post,* August 11, 1983.
2. *In the Matter of Charles P. Osborne,* 294A.2d 372, 1972.
3. President's Commission for the Study of Ethical Problems in Medicine and Biomedical and Behavioral Research, *Making Health Care Decisions* vol. 1 (Washington, DC: Government Printing Office, 1982).
4. Ibid., vol. 3, 201.
5. Jay Katz, "Informed Consent—A Fairy Tale," *University of Pittsburgh Law Review 39* (Winter 1977): 137–174.
6. "Breast Cancer Law Opposed in Richmond," *Washington Post,* August 12, 1983.
7. Margaret Keller Holmes, "Ghost Surgery," *Bulletin of the New York Academy of Medicine 56,* no. 4 (May 1980): 414.
8. Toby Cohen, "The High Cost of Bad Medicine," *Washington Post,* September 20, 1983.
9. Holmes, "Ghost Surgery," 415.
10. American Medical Association, *Current Opinions of the Judicial Council of the American Medical Association,* 1989.
11. American College of Surgeons, "Statements on Principles," 1989.
12. Martin L. Kempner, "Some Moral Issues Concerning Current Ways of Dealing with Surgical Patients," *Bulletin of the New York Academy of Medicine 55,* no. 1 (1979): 62–68.

10

∞

DEATH AND DYING

Death and dying are fundamental aspects of human existence. Like abortion, the ethical questions involved arouse emotional responses from the public and from many health professionals. Questions about death and dying arise in caring for neonates with severe disabilities whose likelihood of survival is minimal. They arise in caring for terminally ill children or adults, who are often unable to express personal autonomy.

Technology is at the heart of the matter. In the past several decades, technological developments such as renal dialysis, mechanical ventilation, and intensive care units have made it possible, in some cases, to postpone the cessation of life, as traditionally measured. Similar developments permit the survival of neonates who only a decade ago would have died. Sometimes the dilemma is that a person asks the organization to assist in achieving a painfree death. Much has been written about the questions raised by such technology, but few universally accepted courses of action have been identified.

Adding complexity is that these ethical issues are poorly developed in the law. Overtly and patently shortening a patient's life raises obvious ethical and legal questions. Judges and juries are reluctant to convict, however, even when violent means have been used to end the painful life of someone terminally ill.

Chapter 9 noted that the President's Commission recommended a physician–patient relationship that maximizes patient sovereignty, and suggested that the patient participate fully in the decision process. Often, by the time crucial medical decisions must be made, the patient is no longer able to participate effectively. A health services system dedicated to preserving life and staving off death takes over. Typically, the demands of the technological imperative are followed, and all efforts are expended, often to achieve only marginal results. The economic and psychological costs are obvious.

Managers are often ill at ease even discussing death and dying. They are likely to consider decision making about death and dying to be a clinical matter in which they have no role to play. Undoubtedly, physicians must be the prime actors, but the effect of such issues on the organization requires that managers be knowledgeable about them and participate in policy development and implementation. Managers should also be involved in any committee-linked activities.

DEFINING DEATH

Historically, death has been defined as the stoppage of blood circulation and the cessation of circulation-dependent animal and vital functions, such as respiration and pulsation. As technology developed, this definition proved inadequate. Table 5 summarizes various definitions of death. Those based in law and theology provide limited help to contemporary clinicians.

In 1968 a committee at the Harvard Medical School issued criteria defining irreversible coma. This was an important development, but one that raised other problems. The original Harvard criteria were accompanied by a report that stated that the patient's condition can be determined only by a physician, and that when the condition is found to be hopeless, certain steps are recommended:

> Death is declared and *then* the respirator is turned off. The decision to do this and the responsibility for it are to be taken by the physician-in-charge, in consultation with one or more physicians who have been directly involved in the case. It is unsound and undesirable to force the family to make the decision.[1]

This quotation is noteworthy because major changes in society's attitudes and perceptions have occurred in the interval. These developments include stress on patient autonomy as expressed through living wills and natural death acts, involvement of the family in decision making, and efforts to establish institutional ethics committees (IECs). The effect of these changes is to diminish the centrality and primacy of the physician's role.

About the time the Harvard criteria were issued, one of the first court cases dealing with brain death was decided in Virginia.[2] It raised issues of consent, appropriate criteria and process for determining death, conflicts of interest, beneficence, nonmaleficence, and organizational philosophy and managerial ethics. For the purposes of this discussion, however, the determination of death is most important. The physicians sought to use a brain death standard, but they failed to meet the Harvard criteria in two ways: they did not use an electroencephalogram in verifying brain activity, and the respirator was turned off before the patient was pronounced dead. Despite these lapses, the court accepted a brain death definition, thus making legal history.

The Harvard criteria have proved reliable. Nonetheless, several criticisms have been raised. They were summarized by the President's Commission:

> 1. The phrase "irreversible coma" is misleading as applied to the cases at hand. "Coma" is a condition of a living person, and a body without any brain functions is dead and thus *beyond* coma.
> 2. The writers of these (Harvard) criteria did not realize that the spinal cord reflexes actually persist or return quite commonly after the brain has completely and permanently ceased functioning.
> 3. "Unreceptivity" is not amenable to testing in an unresponsive body without consciousness.
> 4. The need adequately to test brainstem reflexes, especially apnea, and to ex-

Table 5. Definition of death

Concept of death	Locus of death	Criteria of death
(Philosophical or theological judgment of the essentially significant change at death)	(Place to look to determine if a person has died)	(Measurements physicians or other officials use to determine whether a person is dead—to be determined by scientific empirical study)
1. Irreversible loss of flow of vital fluids (i.e., the blood and breath)	Heart and lungs	Visual observation of respiration, perhaps with the use of a mirror Feeling of the pulse, possibly supported by electrocardiogram
2. Irreversible loss of the soul from the body	Pineal body (?) (according to Descartes) Respiratory tract?	Observation of breath (?)
3. Irreversible loss of the capacity for bodily integration	Brain	Unreceptivity and unresponsivity No movements or breathing No reflexes (except spinal reflexes) Flat electroencephalogram (to be used as confirmatory evidence) All tests to be repeated 24 hours later (excluded conditions: hypothermia and central nervous system drug depression).
4. Irreversible loss of consciousness or the capacity for social interaction	Probably the neocortex	Electroencephalogram

Note: Death is defined as a complete change in the status of a living entity characterized by the irreversible loss of those characteristics that are essentially significant to it. The possible concepts, loci, and criteria of death are much more complex than the ones given here. These are meant to be simplified models of types of positions being taken in the current debate. It is obvious that those who believe that death means the irreversible loss of the capacity for bodily integration (3) or the irreversible loss of consciousness (4) have no reservations about pronouncing death when the heart and lungs have ceased to function. This is because they are willing to use loss of heart and lung activity as shortcut criteria for death, believing that once heart and lungs have stopped, the brain or neocortex will necessarily stop as well.

Adapted from Veatch, R.M. (1976). *Death, dying, and the biological revolution: Our last quest for responsibility.* New Haven: Yale University Press, p. 53. © Yale University Press. Used with permission. This table has been modified using material from the 1989 second edition.

clude drug and metabolic intoxication as possible causes of coma, are not sufficiently explicit and precise.

5. Although all individuals that meet "Harvard criteria" are dead (irreversible cessation of all functions of the entire brain), there are many individuals who are dead but do not maintain circulation long enough to have a 24-hour observation period.[3]

By mid-1990, 31 states and the District of Columbia had enacted the Uniform Determination of Death Act developed by the National Conference of Commissioners on Uniform State Laws.[4] Forty-six states had updated definitions of death.[5] The Uniform Act includes two alternative definitions of death. One definition uses brain death, defined as irreversible cessation of all functions of the entire brain, including the brain stem. The other definition uses irreversible cessation of circulatory and respiratory functions. The brain death definition is endorsed by the American Academy of Neurology.[6]

As scientific developments permit more sophisticated assessments of a patient's condition, especially prognosis, criteria relying on brain death may be superseded by those incorporating psycho-social factors. Prominent among the criteria proposed is the capacity or potential capacity for social interaction. This definition raises ethical issues, and puts in jeopardy persons who have no capacity for normal social interaction (e.g., people with severe mental retardation). A definition that includes a lack of the potential for social interaction was applied when infants with mental retardation, such as Baby Boy Doe, were allowed to die. Although new federal regulations specifically prohibit applying quality of life criteria to infants with disabilities who have life-threatening medical conditions, there is ample evidence that quality of life criteria are commonly used in decision making for other types of patients.

TERMINATING LIFE

Hospitals have been reluctant to discontinue life support without a specific judicial determination. This reluctance seems to be based more on the fear of legal liability than on a search for the ethically correct action. The leading case is *In re Quinlan*. Karen Ann Quinlan was 21 years old in mid-1975 when she became comatose after ingesting an overdose of alcohol and tranquilizers. The New Jersey Supreme Court overturned a trial court ruling and permitted Karen's father to be appointed her guardian.[7] The court authorized Mr. Quinlan to discontinue all extraordinary measures to sustain life if the family and physicians agreed that there was no reasonable possibility that Karen would emerge from her vegetative state and if there was consultation with the hospital ethics committee. This is one of the earliest enunciations of a role for ethics committees, and it served as a stimulus for New Jersey hospitals to establish such committees. In the context of the opinion, it is clear, however, that the court intended that the committee would be a prognosis committee, a rather different role from that which ethics committees have assumed.

After Mr. Quinlan ordered the respirator disconnected, the physicians weaned Karen successfully and she breathed unaided. She was discharged to a nursing home, where she remained until her death in mid-1985. When she died, she weighed 66 pounds and her body was locked in a fetal position.

In addition to New Jersey, courts in Massachusetts and New York have been especially active in cases like *Quinlan*. Such cases have been brought either by next of kin seeking to regain control from the health services organization, or by managers seeking protection from legal claims. Not all such cases have followed *Quinlan*. Some patients have received continued treatment even when there was no reasonable likelihood of benefit. In other situations, painful treatment that would have been of little benefit was withheld. With guidance from the courts, health services organizations are attempting to solve the problem of when it is appropriate to discontinue life support. The courts are a necessary arbiter in settling legal questions that arise, especially when there is dissonance between the ethics of the persons and the ethics of the organizations involved. By defining limits of the law, court decisions are important in aiding persons and organizations to develop and refine their ethic.

CARING FOR INFANTS WITH DISABILITIES

Babies Doe

Recent developments with ethical dimensions similar to those in *Quinlan* include the Baby Doe cases. The name derives from court proceedings in several states in the early 1980s. All of these cases were similar to the case of Baby Boy Doe, whose situation was described in Chapter 1. All involved parents who decided to forego life-sustaining treatment of their newborn infants who had treatable genetic anomalies. Publicity surrounding the subsequent deaths of two such infants prompted the Department of Health and Human Services (HHS) to issue regulations in April, 1982, prohibiting hospitals that receive federal funds from withholding life-sustaining treatment from infants with disabilities. Authority for this action was claimed in Section 504 of the Rehabilitation Act of 1973, which prohibits discrimination on the basis of handicap. The regulations were challenged by health services organizations on procedural grounds and an injunction suspending implementation was issued. Another attempt to promulgate a modified version of the regulations followed in 1983. Like the first regulations, they mandated telephone hotlines to report alleged cases of withholding life-sustaining treatment from seriously ill newborns. By law, signs with information about the need to treat such newborns had to be posted. For providers, the hotlines were the most hated and controversial requirement. Opponents claimed that the regulations turned providers into spies and stool pigeons. An important modification in the 1983 revisions was that impossible or futile acts or therapies that merely prolonged the dying of an infant born terminally ill were not required. Those opposing the regulations successfully obtained judicial relief preventing implementation.

In June, 1985, the U.S. Supreme Court agreed to hear a Justice Department appeal of a lower court decision that invalidated the Baby Doe regulations. This was surprising, because the actions of Congress and HHS had made moot the need for the first regulations. Nonetheless, in June, 1986, the Supreme Court agreed with the lower court in an opinion that struck down the Baby Doe rules. It agreed that Section 504 of the Rehabilitation Act of 1973 did not empower HHS to force hospitals to treat infants with severe disabilities over the objections of their parents. The Supreme Court's decision displeased some disability advocacy groups, who claimed that there are major enforcement problems with the Child Abuse Amendments of 1984, both procedurally and as the result of a basic antihandicap bias on the parts of physicians and child protective services agencies. They contended that these biases will result in a decision not to treat in large numbers of cases.

Child Abuse Amendments

The original controversy surrounding Baby Boy Doe prompted Congress to deal directly with the question of newborns with serious disabilities. The Child Abuse Amendments of 1984 (P.L. 98-457) were signed into law October 9, 1984. They establish treatment and reporting guidelines for care of newborns with severe disabilities. Withholding "medically indicated treatment" from infants with disabilities is illegal except when

> in the treating physician's(s') reasonable medical judgment (i) the infant is chronically and irreversibly comatose; (ii) the provision of such treatment would merely prolong dying, not be effective in ameliorating or correcting all of the infant's life-threatening conditions, or otherwise be futile in terms of survival of the infant; or (iii) the provision of such treatment would be virtually futile in terms of the survival of the infant and the treatment itself under such circumstances would be inhumane.[8]

Treatment is defined to include appropriate nonextraordinary care, such as nutrition and hydration, as well as medication.[9]

Under the law, appropriate health services organizations must designate persons who will report suspected problems to state child protective services agencies. The agencies coordinate and consult with those persons and, after notification of cases of suspected medical neglect, may initiate legal action.

Infant Care Review Committees

P.L. 98-457 directs HHS to encourage establishment of infant care review committees (ICRC) within health facilities, especially those with tertiary level neonatal units, to:

> (1) educate hospital personnel and families of disabled infants with life-threatening conditions; (2) recommend institutional policies and guidelines concerning the

withholding of medically indicated treatment from infants with life-threatening conditions; and (3) offer counsel and review in cases involving infants with life-threatening conditions.[10]

In effect, this is a type of specialized ethics committee that will provide information and education, recommend institutional policies and guidelines, and offer counsel and review. This individualized hospital effort should produce higher-quality results. The guidelines are clear that although HHS considers it prudent to establish an ICRC, the decision rests with the organization.

Many groups, including the American Medical Association (AMA), the American Hospital Association (AHA), and various medical specialty associations, objected vociferously to the original regulations and led the fight to block implementation. The Child Abuse Amendments and regulations, however, are supported by health services trade associations covering the gamut of institutional and personal providers, as well as specialized groups. In fact, such associations were instrumental in developing both the law and the regulations, their support was reported in the background information provided in the proposed rules issued by HHS in late 1984. The new law was enthusiastically backed by the AHA, and hospitals are likely to have few philosophical problems complying with it.[11]

WITHDRAWING TREATMENT

Although in theory patients retain the right to determine what care they receive and when it will be discontinued, treatment processes for institutionalized patients, even those who are alert, often become psychologically and physically overwhelming. The processes and the persons who apply them dominate; the patient quickly loses control. Patients (or their representatives) may have to bring legal action to exercise their autonomy.

Instructions from the Formerly Competent

Constance Emerson has lived a full life, but at 92 she is confined to a nursing home. Three years ago she fell and suffered a cerebral hemorrhage. Her mental faculties remain impaired even after extensive therapy. Earlier in life she was active in the community. She worked as a volunteer at Homer House, a noted settlement house, where she led development of educational programs for children of working mothers.

After the injury, Mrs. Emerson's husband cared for her until the deterioration of his own health made it impossible for him to continue to do so. Mrs. Emerson has long had diabetes. She requires a special diet and insulin. She eats only soft foods or liquids, and is bedridden, blind, and deaf. She has occasional respiratory infections that respond well to treatment. Her heart is strong. Except for mild arthritis, she has no pain. She sometimes recognizes her husband when he visits, but her speech is often unintelligible.

Three years before her accident, Mrs. Emerson gave a talk on the miseries of prolonging life for the dying elderly. Having seen the agony of deterioration in her relatives, she made an eloquent plea for a "dignified and simple way to choose death." She showed the manuscript to Mr. Emerson and mentioned publishing it, but had not. Mr. Emerson now fears speaking to her about what she had written or how she feels about her life because she might infer that he wants her to die. Their son visits her weekly and states they should not disturb the care she is receiving.[12]

This case illustrates the ethical problems associated with caring for infirm elderly people. The care provided Mrs. Emerson maintains her, but nothing can be done to reverse the brain damage she suffered. She is not terminally ill. The care Mrs. Emerson requires and receives is ordinary for her general condition. (The concepts of ordinary and extraordinary used as criteria to judge whether to withhold or withdraw treatment are discussed later.) There is some evidence as to what Mrs. Emerson thought about other people in conditions similar to hers, but that information is several years old. Her current wishes are not known, and it is impossible to determine them because of her mental state. Even if she were able to express her wishes about continuing her life, or had some written directive that could be used, she could not direct the organization to assist her in ending her life. Because she is not terminally ill, discontinuing treatment is inappropriate.

A new development, called *assisted suicide,* which can be classified as a form of voluntary, active euthanasia is discussed below. An underlying assumption for assisted suicide is that the person contemplating suicide be mentally competent. This requirement would deny the option to Mrs. Emerson.

It is instructive to apply the last definition of death in Table 5 to the case of Mrs. Emerson. Is she "alive" if a criterion of capacity for social interaction is applied? The case notes that she "sometimes recognizes her husband when he visits." Whether she has the capacity for social interaction is something that could be determined. If it were determined that she is not capable of social interaction, this definition would allow her to die by withholding antibiotics or insulin. Whether this could, or should, be done absent an advance directive is another question. Considering the facts in this case, however, the only ethical action is to continue hydration, nutrition, and medication.

ADVANCE DIRECTIVES

Living Wills

The living will was developed as a way for persons to retain control of their lives when they may be unable to participate in decision-making processes. The concept of living wills is several decades old and has been publicized exten-sively by an organization called Concern for Dying. The words *living* and *will* seem contradictory. A traditional will is the legal mechanism by which a per-son's wishes are carried out after the person's death. Living wills allow persons unable to communicate with caregivers to express their wishes about treatment. A primary function is to allow patients to limit what is done for and to them, and to control the technological imperative whether or not it will ultimately benefit the patient or is wanted by the patient. A sample living will is shown in Figure 10. Unless legislation specifically upholding living wills exists (as dis-cussed in the next section), living wills have no legal status; patients must rely on the willingness of caregivers to accept such documents. The sample living will form shown in Figure 10 was developed by a private organization. It is unlikely to meet specific state requirements, but could be useful in states in which no statutes exist.

Natural Death Act Statutes

Public interest in living wills and the publicity given to cases in which more treatment was provided than many people would want led to rapid state enact-ment of natural death acts, or death with dignity laws. By early 1983, 14 states recognized living wills. The form used in Virginia is shown as Figure 11. By 1985, 35 states and the District of Columbia had laws recognizing living wills. By 1990, the number of states had increased to 42.[13]

The laws generally recognize a patient's right to instruct physicians to withhold or withdraw life-sustaining procedures. The patient must complete the required forms, which, when completed properly, are legally binding. The laws tend to be drafted narrowly, and typically apply only to situations in which it has been medically determined that the patient who signed the declaration is dying and has no prospect of recovery. In some states, the decision must be reaffirmed when patients know they have a terminal illness. Some laws provide for penalties against caregivers and the organization when instructions are ig-nored.[14] In addition to the statutes, appeals court and state supreme court deci-sions affect the way the laws are interpreted and life-sustaining treatment is withheld or withdrawn.

These laws solve some of the issues of control (autonomy), patient role, and to an extent, organizational and provider efforts to comply with the pa-tient's wishes. There continue to be problems, such as determining the patient's mental status, establishing the presence of a terminal illness, and determining whether the patient comprehends the effect of what is being done. Of course, the ethical dilemma remains for organizations in situations in which the patient has not met the provisions of the statute or the state has no statute.

Durable Power of Attorney

An increasingly common example of surrogate decision making regarding life continuation decisions is the durable power of attorney for health care. The law

To My Family, My Physician, My Lawyer, And All Others Whom It May Concern

Death is as much a reality as birth, growth, and aging—it is the one certainty of life. In anticipation of decisions that may have to be made about my own dying and as an expression of my right to refuse treatment, I _____, being of sound mind, make this statement of
(print name)
my wishes and instructions concerning treatment.

By means of this document, which I intend to be legally binding, I direct my physician and other care providers, my family, and any surrogate designated by me or appointed by a court, to carry out my wishes. If I become unable, by reason of physical or mental incapacity, to make decisions about my medical care, let this document provide the guidance and authority needed to make any and all such decisions.

If I am permanently unconscious or there is no reasonable expectation of my recovery from a seriously incapacitating or lethal illness or condition, I do not wish to be kept alive by artificial means. I request that I be given all care necessary to keep me comfortable and free of pain, even if pain-relieving medications may hasten my death, and I direct that no life-sustaining treatment be provided except as I or my surrogate specifically authorize.

This request may appear to place a heavy responsibility upon you, but by making this decision according to my strong convictions, I intend to ease that burden. I am acting after careful consideration and with understanding of the consequences of your carrying out my wishes. *List optional specific provisions in the space below.*

How to Use Your Living Will

The Living Will should clearly state your preferences about life-sustaining treatment. You may wish to add specific statements to the Living Will in the space provided for that purpose. Such statements might concern:
- Cardiopulmonary resuscitation
- Artificial or invasive measures for providing nutrition and hydration
- Kidney dialysis
- Mechanical or artificial respiration
- Blood transfusion
- Surgery (such as amputation)
- Antibiotics

You may also wish to indicate any preferences you may have about such matters as dying at home.

Important Points to Remember

- Sign and date your Living Will.
- Your two witnesses should not be blood relatives, your spouse, potential beneficiaries of your estate or your health care proxy.
- Discuss your Living Will with your doctors; and give them copies of your Living Will for inclusion in your medical file, so they will know whom to contact in the event something happens to you.
- Make photo copies of your Living Will and give them to anyone who may be making decisions for you if you are unable to make them yourself.
- Place the original in a safe, accessible place, so that it can be located if needed—not in a safe deposit box.
- Look over your Living Will periodically (at least every five years), initial and redate it so that it will be clear that your wishes have not changed.

Figure 10. A sample living will. (From Concern for Dying, 250 W. 57th St., New York, NY. Reprinted with permission.)

Written Natural Death Act Declaration

A declaration executed pursuant to this article may, but need not, be in one of the following forms, and may include other specific directions including, but not limited to, a designation of another person to make the treatment decision for the declarant should he be (i) diagnosed as suffering from a terminal condition and (ii) comatose, incompetent or otherwise mentally or physically incapable of communication. Should any other specific directions be held to be invalid, such invalidity shall not affect the delcaration.

Declaration made this _____ day of _____ (month, year).

I, _____ ,

wilfully and voluntarily make known my desire and do hereby declare:

CHOOSE ONLY ONE OF THE NEXT TWO
PARAGRAPHS AND CROSS THROUGH THE OTHER

If at any time I should have a terminal condition and my attending physician has determined that there can be no recovery from such condition, my death is imminent, and I am comatose, incompetent or otherwise mentally or physically incapable of communication, I designate .... to make a decision on my behalf as to whether life prolonging procedures shall be withheld or withdrawn. In the event that my designee decides that such procedures should be withheld or withdrawn, I wish to be permitted to die naturally with only the administration of medication or the performance of any medical procedure deemed necessary to provide me with comfort care or to alleviate pain.

If at any time I should have a terminal condition and my attending physician has determined that there can be no recovery from such condition and my death is imminent, where the application of life-prolonging procedures would serve only to artificially prolong the dying process, I direct that such procedures be withheld or withdrawn, and that I be permitted to die naturally with only the administration of medication or the performance of any medical procedure deemed necessary to provide me with comfort care or to alleviate pain.

In the absence of my ability to give directions regarding the use of such life-prolonging procedures, it is my intention that this declaration shall be honored by my family and physician as the final expression of my legal right to refuse medical or surgical treatment and accept the consequences of such refusal.

I understand the full import of this declaration and I am emotionally and mentally competent to make this declaration.

_____
(Signed)
The declarant is known to me and I believe him or her to be of sound mind.

_____
Witness

_____
Witness

Figure 11. Suggested form of Written Natural Death Act Declaration adopted by the State of Virginia. (From *Code of Virginia* 1950, 1990 Cumulative Supplement vol. 7A. Title 54.1, Article 8, section 2984, 197–198.)

has long recognized powers of attorney as a way for persons to delegate to another certain authority to act for them. A power of attorney is durable when the grant of authority extends beyond the time when the person granting it becomes incapacitated. By mid-1990, 25 states and the District of Columbia had statutes extending durable powers of attorney to health care decisions. Eighteen of these states and the District of Columbia specifically allow agents to make decisions regarding withdrawing or withholding life support. A number of other states rely on court decisions, attorneys' general opinions, or special attention to this issue in their natural death act statutes.[15] A sample durable power of attorney form is shown in Figure 12. Like the living will form in Figure 10, this form is unlikely to meet specific state requirements, but could be useful in states without statutes.

Do-Not-Resuscitate (DNR) Orders

Many patients do not have living wills, or have not signed advance directives that meet the requirements of a natural death act. This makes it particularly important that the organization have policies and processes that address questions about resuscitating terminally ill patients and patients for whom life continuation decisions must be made (e.g., patients in persistent vegetative states [PVS]). Many organizations have adopted do-not-resuscitate (DNR) policies that affirm the right of patients (or a surrogate, as appropriate) to provide direction to their caregivers regarding the aggressiveness of life-saving efforts. The DNR policy should identify which chemical and mechanical technologies are included, and which technologies will be applied to which patients.

A study at three Houston teaching hospitals showed that DNR orders are applied inconsistently.[16] The hospitals in the study did not have DNR policies. The study found that some DNR patients continued to undergo chemotherapy and surgery, and were admitted to the intensive care unit. At the other extreme, some DNR patients received inadequate hydration and nutrition. Staff are often confused about what care to give DNR patients, perhaps because they personally disagree with decisions to keep some patients alive. The study found that in 10% of the cases, no decision had been reached on whether to try to keep the patient alive. This indicates that attempts to decide about resuscitation in advance of crises are failing in a number of cases. In most no decision cases, the subject of DNR had not even been brought up with the patient or family. Other studies of DNR orders report similar findings.[17] Another dimension of DNR orders has to do with whether they are written equitably for patients with different diseases but similar prognoses. A study reported in 1989 found that DNR orders are much more likely to be written for patients with AIDS or inoperable lung cancer than for patients with other diseases with equally poor prognoses, such as cirrhosis or heart failure. Reasons for the differences were not reported by the researchers.[18]

Durable Power of Attorney
for Health Care Decisions

To effect my wishes, I designate _____,
residing at _____ (Phone #) _____,
(or if he or she shall for any reason fail to act, _____
(Phone #) _____, residing at _____)
as my health care surrogate—that is, my attorney-in-fact regarding any and all
health care decisions to be made for me, including the decision to refuse life-
sustaining treatment—if I am unable to make such decisions myself. This power
shall remain effective during and not be affected by my subsequent illness, disability or incapacity. My surrogate shall have authority to interpret my Living
Will, and shall make decisions about my health care as specified in my instructions or, when my wishes are not clear, as the surrogate believes to be in my best
interests. I release and agree to hold harmless my health care surrogate from any
and all claims whatsoever arising from decisions made in good faith in the exercise of this power.

I sign this document knowingly, voluntarily, and after careful delibera-
tion, this _____ day of _____, 19_____.

_____
(signature)

Address _____

Witness _____
Printed Name _____
Address _____
_____

Witness _____
Printed Name _____
Address _____
_____

I do hereby certify that the within document was executed and acknowledged before me by the principal this
_____ day of _____, 19_____.

_____

Notary Public

Copies of this document have been
given to:

The Durable Power of Attorney for Health Care

This optional feature permits you to name a surrogate decision maker (also
known as a proxy, health agent or attorney-in-fact), someone to make health care
decisions on your behalf if you lose that ability. As this person should act according to your preferences and in your best interests, you should select this person
with care and make certain that he or she knows what your wishes are and about
your Living Will.

You should not name someone who is a witness to your Living Will. You
may want to name an alternate agent in case the first person you select is unable or
unwilling to serve. If you do name a surrogate decision maker, the form must be
notarized. (It is a good idea to notarize the document in any case.)

Figure 12. A sample durable power of attorney for health care decisions. (From Concern for
Dying, 250 W. 57th St., New York, NY. Reprinted with permission.)

Veatch considers the more important problem to be one of failing to undertake treatment because the physician assumes it is not in a patient's interests, or because the physician believes the patient would not want it.[19] Late in 1990, efforts to achieve patient participation in and direction of their health care decisions received a substantial boost when Congress included provisions of Senate Bill 1766, the Patient Self Determination Act of 1989, in the Omnibus Budget Reconciliation Act of 1990 (P.L. 101-508). The provisions require Medicare providers to provide adults receiving care with written information about their rights, under state law, to accept or refuse medical or surgical treatment and their right to formulate advance directives, and to provide adults with the provider's written policies concerning implementing these rights. The provider must document in the medical record whether a patient has an advance medical directive. Providers must also educate their staffs and the community on issues concerning advance directives. Such actions do not consider the autonomy of the patient—either as an independent decision maker or as an involved participant. These findings suggest that there are major ethical problems involving DNR orders for terminally ill patients in hospitals.

Summary

It has been suggested that widespread use of natural death act declarations might encourage systematic rationing of health care to the elderly. If a right to die becomes a duty to die, the living will and its progeny, the natural death act declaration, will have become a Frankenstein monster. Indeed, the suggestion by then Governor Lamm of Colorado, as well as officials at HHS, that the elderly should be required to have living wills raised a storm of protest. Regardless of the true motives behind such statements, such suggestions are usually seen as being economically motivated.

The legislative trend toward formal means by which patients are involved in decision making about death reflects changed attitudes in society. A survey conducted by the American Board of Family Practice found that over 50% of the general public and 64% of family physicians think that requests by the patient and the patient's family that the patient be allowed to die should be honored.[20] A recent study of hospitals showed that two thirds have a formal policy on advance directives. Of these, however, most put the burden on the patient (or the patient's surrogates) to tell them or the physician that such a document exists. Only 4% have policies that ask all patients at the time they are admitted whether they have advance directives.[21]

The organization must be alert to the ethical problems regarding advance directives, which may be present whether or not a natural death act statute has been enacted or a living will signed. Health services organizations and their managers must address these issues prospectively, and develop policies that respect patients' wishes, consistent with the organizational philosophy.

EUTHANASIA

The terms *natural death* or *death with dignity* should not be confused with the term *euthanasia*. The first two terms mean that a patient's life is not extended artificially and that life-sustaining treatment can be withheld or withdrawn at the request of patients or surrogates empowered to do so. The word *euthanasia* comes from the Greek *eu*, meaning good or easy, and *thanatos*, meaning death. If used accurately and in its correct historical context, it describes situations in which someone is cared for in a manner that makes an inevitable death as free of pain as possible. No artificial means need be used to extend life. The term *euthanasia*, however, is often incorrectly used to refer to situations in which active steps are taken to cause someone's death (e.g., mercy killing). This use blurs important distinctions. Assisting persons to have a painfree death is helping them to die naturally and with dignity.

Morphia Somnolence

Henrietta Morrow was diagnosed as having inoperable cancer 18 months ago. Chemotherapy was attempted, but it had no effect on the disease. The lymph system had spread the cancer throughout her body, and Morrow was in severe pain. Initially, she received care at home from nurses from the local hospice. Now, however, the disease had worsened and she could not receive adequate care at home. She had become an inpatient at the hospice. Her life expectancy was estimated at less than 3 months.

In addition to nutrition, hydration, and other comfort care, Morrow received a variant of Bromton's cocktail (a mixture of water, lemon extract, syrup, cocaine, morphine, 95% ethanol, and phenothiazine). (The original Bromton's cocktail included heroin, but heroin cannot be legally dispensed in the United States.) As the disease progressed, the proportion of morphine was increased to deal more effectively with the pain. The nursing staff raised with the hospice's medical director their concern about the depressant effect the morphine would have on Morrow's respiratory system. They felt that they risked depressing it to the point where they might actively cause her death. The concern was expressed within both a legal and an ethical context. The medical director assured them there were no legal problems, and described the ethical considerations. They included: ordinary compared with extraordinary care, active and passive euthanasia, voluntary versus involuntary euthanasia, and the principle of double effect.

Ordinary Versus Extraordinary Care

To hasten or bring about death by increasing the proportion of morphine beyond the level needed to control pain would be euthanasia, an act that is both unethical and illegal. To continue chemotherapy would be considered extraordinary care for someone like Morrow. Comfort care and the pain relief provided by the Bromton's cocktail also represent ordinary care. Historically, hydration and nutrition were considered ordinary care. However, whether such care represents extraordinary or ordinary treatment is now a hotly contested issue. Under the principle of nonmaleficence, the distinction is as follows:

> Ordinary means are all medicines, treatments, and operations which offer reasonable hope of benefit and which can be obtained and used without excessive expense, pain, or other inconvenience. Extraordinary means are all medicines, treatments, and operations which cannot be obtained or used without excessive expense, pain, or inconvenience, or which, if used, would not offer a reasonable hope of benefit.[22]

Ordinary and extraordinary should not be interpreted to mean usual and unusual, respectively. Doing so leads to confusion, primarily because of the variation even among similar hospitals as to treatments considered usual or unusual. Usual emergency treatment provided in a shock trauma unit is quite different from that provided in a community hospital. The measure is the hope of benefit as compared with excessiveness of expense, pain, or other inconvenience. Absent hope of benefit, any medicine, treatments, or operations could be considered extraordinary. If there is hope of benefit, use of the same medicines, treatments, and operations may not be excessive.

It has been suggested that the terms *proportionate* and *disproportionate* are clearer and more descriptive than the terms *ordinary* and *extraordinary*. The criteria for measuring proportionate and disproportionate care are very similar to those for ordinary and extraordinary, but are stated somewhat differently. The type of treatment to be used, its degree of complexity or risk, its cost, and the appropriateness of using it are studied and compared with the results that can be expected, taking into account the state of sick persons and their physical and moral resources.[23] A simplified statement summarizing the concepts of ordinary/extraordinary or proportionate/disproportionate is: "Does the benefit justify the burden?"

Applying these criteria in the case of Mrs. Emerson, who needed special diets, insulin, and occasional antibiotics, results in the conclusion that nothing being done for her is extraordinary. All of the care she is receiving offers reasonable hope of benefit without excessive expense, pain, or inconvenience. The reasonable hope of benefit is not based on any expectation that she will regain her former mental and physical condition, but that she will have the life of someone 92 years old who has experienced head trauma.

Active or Passive Euthanasia

The case of Henrietta Morrow raises questions about the concept of euthanasia. Do the actions there constitute active or passive, voluntary or involuntary euthanasia? Active euthanasia occurs when the patient's death is purposely hastened. Giving Morrow an overdose of morphine would represent active euthanasia, which is criminal homicide. Passive euthanasia occurs when the patient is allowed to die and no extraordinary means are used to prolong life, or when extraordinary means for prolonging life are withdrawn and the patient is allowed to die. Withholding or withdrawing life-sustaining treatment does not preclude comfort care, pain control, and nutrition and hydration. In some situations, it is argued that artificially provided nutrition and hydration constitute extraordinary (disproportionate) care, however.

Voluntary or Involuntary Euthanasia

The terms *voluntary* and *involuntary* euthanasia refer to patient wishes in decisions about treatment. There is no information as to whether Morrow has been told that increasing quantities of morphine might shorten her life. While it is reasonable to assume that she prefers to be painfree despite the other effects of the morphine, an organization that emphasizes autonomy will to the greatest extent possible involve the competent patient in decision making about all treatment, including pain control.

Principle of Double Effect

The Morrow case also raises the issue of the moral precept of double effect. Like the concept of ordinary and extraordinary care, double effect is a subset of the principle of nonmaleficence.

> The principle of double effect specifies four conditions that must be satisfied for an act with both a good and a bad effect to be justified: (1) The action itself (independent of its consequences) must not be intrinsically wrong (it must be morally good or at least morally neutral). (2) The agent must intend only the good effect and not the bad effect. The bad effect can be foreseen, tolerated, and permitted but not be intended. . . . (3) The bad effect must not be a *means* to the end of bringing about the good effect; that is, the good effect must be achieved directly by the action and not by way of the bad effect. (4) The good result must outweigh the evil permitted; that is, there must be proportionality or a favorable balance between the good and bad effects of the action.[24]

The principle of double effect allows ethical use of morphine, even in increasing quantities, to ease Morrow's pain.

SUICIDE AND THE ORGANIZATION

The *Bouvia* Case

A case highlighting several of the concepts described above began in California in late 1983. Elizabeth Bouvia entered county-owned Riverside General Hospital and asked that the staff aid her in fasting until she died. Bouvia has cerebral palsy. She is unable to move and requires assistance in all physical activities. Bouvia entered the hospital in order to receive the hygienic care and drugs necessary to facilitate a painless death by starvation. Initially, Riverside General Hospital wanted to discharge her, but was prevented from doing so by a court injunction. To ensure adequate nutrition, hospital staff inserted a nasogastric feeding tube, allegedly against Bouvia's wishes. She asserted that she had reached a competent and rational decision, one her lawyer argued was protected by the constitutional right to privacy and self-determination. Her mental competence was confirmed by all of the psychiatrists who examined her.

In a hearing on the issue of whether the hospital had to assist Bouvia in her suicide, the court ruled that "despite her right to commit suicide, which is not illegal in California, she could not ask society in the person of the hospital staff to help her because she was not a terminal patient."[25] It is important to note that aiding and abetting a suicide in California is a criminal act. The court distinguished people who are terminally ill from persons, such as Bouvia, who have severe health problems but are not terminally ill. In January, 1984, the California Supreme Court refused to hear Bouvia's appeal.[26]

The decision permitted the hospital to force feed Bouvia. She was discharged from Riverside General April 7, 1984, and was hospitalized in Tijuana, Mexico.[27] The press reported that she had reconsidered the decision to end her life and would return to the United States for medical treatment. Her lawyer maintained, however, that she still wished to die, despite the fact that she had been accepted for care somewhere in California on the condition that she not stop eating.[28]

After a year in the new institution and a subsequent stay of several months at an acute care hospital, where a morphine pump for pain control was installed, Bouvia was admitted to Los Angeles County-High Desert Hospital in late 1985. As at Riverside General Hospital, and against her wishes, the staff inserted a permanent feeding tube to provide nutrition. Court action by Bouvia initially resulted in the court's refusal to order discontinuation of the force feeding. On appeal, however, the case was remanded, with instructions to consider her request further. As a result, tube feeding was ordered discontinued and she was discharged. Her attorney stated: "She's promised to continue to eat her liquid diet. I know she would welcome death . . . but she has renounced (suicide)."[29] In May, 1986, she was hospitalized at Los Angeles County-University of Southern California Medical Center, where she received treatment for chronic pain.[30] In June, 1986, the California Supreme Court upheld a lower court decision allowing her to end her life by refusing forced feeding (at the time she was accepting a liquid diet). The hospital had argued that removal of the tube would amount to an official endorsement of suicide.[31] Since that time, Bouvia has shunned publicity.

In addition to highlighting the problems of the nonterminally ill, the

Bouvia case clearly delineates the clash between organizational philosophy (here with both ethical and legal justification) and patient autonomy. Bouvia's problem was not that the institutions in which she was treated refused to discharge her, but that she had great difficulty finding a facility that would admit her. Institutions that agreed to admit her insisted on doing everything they could to maintain or improve her physical condition—thus the forced feeding. Several state courts have specifically addressed this issue. By late 1989, 16 states permitted withholding or withdrawing tube feeding; 3 states prohibit such actions under certain circumstances.[32]

The *Henninger* Case

It is useful to contrast the *Bouvia* case with a case decided by the New York Supreme Court (the appellate division in New York state). There, 85-year-old G. Ross Henninger suffered from confusion, depression, and irritability, and was hospitalized for treatment of fever and infection. These conditions were compounded by the recovering stroke victim's arthritis, heart disease, and hardening of the arteries. The justice stated he would not "go against (Henninger's) wishes and order this 85-year-old person to be operated on, or be force fed, or to be restrained for the rest of his natural life."[33] The decision was issued following a hearing in which attorneys for Henninger and the nursing home in which he lived petitioned the court to determine the legality of the nursing home allowing him to starve to death. Henninger died the day following the decision.

The *Cruzan* Case

One of the most important cases of the 1990s is the case of a young woman named Nancy Cruzan, who sustained severe injuries (including cerebral contusions compounded by significant anoxia) in an automobile accident in 1983. Initially, Cruzan was in a coma, but she progressed to an unconscious state, and was subsequently diagnosed as being in a PVS. To ease feeding and further her recovery, a gastrostomy tube was inserted to provide hydration and nutrition. When it became apparent that Cruzan had virtually no chance of regaining her mental faculties, her parents asked employees at the Missouri state hospital that was providing her care to terminate artificial hydration and nutrition. The employees refused to do so without court approval. The parents successfully sought court authorization from a state trial court. The trial court found that a person in Cruzan's condition had a fundamental right under the state and federal constitutions to refuse or direct the withdrawal of "death prolonging procedures." The decision was appealed, and the Supreme Court of Missouri reversed the trial court.

The Supreme Court of Missouri recognized that a right to refuse treatment is embodied in the common law doctrine of informed consent, but did not consider it applicable to this case. It also declined to read into the state constitution a broad right to privacy that would support an unrestricted right to refuse treatment, and expressed doubt that the Constitution embodied such a right. The court then decided that the state living will statute embodied a state policy strongly favoring preservation of life, and that Cruzan's statements to her housemate that she would not want to continue her life unless she could live "halfway normally" were unreliable for the purpose of determining her intent.[34] It rejected the argument that her parents were entitled to order the termination of her medical treatment, concluding that no person can make that choice on behalf of an incompetent person in the absence of the formalities required by the living will statute or clear and convincing evidence of the patient's wishes.

Upon petition for certiorari, the U.S. Supreme Court agreed to review the case, and to determine whether Cruzan had a right under the Constitution that would require the hospital to withdraw life-sustaining treatment under these circumstances. On June 25, 1990, the Supreme Court affirmed the Missouri decision.[35] The Court found that the Constitution does not forbid Missouri to require that evidence of an incompetent person's wishes as to the withdrawal of life-sustaining treatment be proved by clear and convincing evidence. The Court distinguished the rights of competent persons, who, the Court assumed, have a constitutionally protected right to refuse life-saving hydration and nutrition, from the rights of incompetent persons. It noted that while Missouri had in effect recognized that under certain circumstances a surrogate may act for the patient in electing to withdraw hydration and nutrition and thus cause death, the state has established a procedural safeguard to ensure that the surrogate's action conforms as closely as possible to the wishes expressed by the patient while competent. The Court went on to grant broad latitude to the states in their efforts to protect and preserve human life; it recognized their right to require a standard that "clear and convincing evidence" be presented as to the person's intentions regarding life continuation decisions. It also noted that the state is entitled to guard against potential abuses by surrogates who may not act to protect the interests of the patient. In addition, the state may properly decline to make judgments about the quality of a particular person's life, and simply assert an unqualified interest in the preservation of human life to be weighed against the constitutionally protected interests of the individual. *Cruzan* makes it clear that the Court is unwilling to extend to incompetent persons the same constitutional right of self-determination that is available to competent persons. The Court found it appropriate that the state establish procedures and safeguards to be used in such decisions. The opinion seemed to give considerable weight to the fact that there was a law, and that the state had considered how such matters should be considered and solved. The Court made no attempt to outline the limits of the range of actions that a legislature could take.

In November, 1990, Ms. Cruzan's parents were granted a second hearing in state court, which the state of Missouri did not oppose. New evidence convinced the judge that Nancy Cruzan would not have wanted to live in a PVS. On

December 14, 1990, he ordered the feeding tube removed. Antieuthanasia groups unsuccessfully sought to intervene, and Cruzan died of dehydration December 26, 1990, 8 years after her accident.[36]

Implications

The *Cruzan* case is important in providing guidance to the states as to acceptable approaches to solving life-continuation decisions. *Cruzan* makes it clear that the states have both the authority and the responsibility to legislate an acceptable process to address such situations, and the Court has granted broad latitude to the states to develop their laws. Health services organizations will draw their guidance from their state's laws. In addition, they carry a special burden—that of advising patients as to their rights under state law to prepare an advance directive. The organization must go beyond informing and assisting the patient and actually ensure that that guidance becomes part of the medical record and is actually applied in the process of care. The fact that research shows that most hospitals put the burden of preparing advance directives on patients and that virtually none advises patients about their use, indicates that much work remains to be done. Health services organizations must meet that challenge as part of their commitment to the principles of respect for persons, beneficence, and nonmaleficence.

Cases such as *Henninger* and *Cruzan* have fueled the debate about whether health services organizations and their clinical staff are obligated to administer food and water artificially to patients who are terminally ill or in PVS. For some patients who must be sedated or restrained to tolerate tube feedings or intravenous lines, the burdens of receiving care are significant, and it must be questioned whether care in this context is always required.[37] Another way to state the issue is that for this type of patient, providing life-sustaining food and water may represent extraordinary (disproportionate) care, although under usual circumstances, nutrition and hydration represent ordinary (proportionate) care.

Whether feeding and hydrating patients who are terminally ill or in PVS is or should ever be considered extraordinary (disproportionate) care will be challenged by many. The AMA, however, has resolved the issue. In March, 1986, its Council on Ethical and Judicial Affairs issued a statement that it is not unethical for physicians to "discontinue all means of life-prolonging medical treatment" from terminally ill or irreversibly comatose patients. These treatments are defined to include medication and artificially or technologically supplied respiration, nutrition, or hydration. ". . . the physician should determine whether the benefits of treatment outweigh its burdens. At all times, the dignity of the patient should be maintained."[38] Protests were made by those who fear that the new policy might cause physicians to discontinue nutrition when they consider it in the patient's best interests even though patients may believe their interests are furthered by being fed, but are unable to communicate this decision. Others object to the new ethic by noting that failure to provide food and water is repugnant because it runs counter to human instincts.

Regardless of the direction the debate takes at the theoretical level, an ethic must be applied at the bedside. What is the right action for a particular patient? Here, the debate begins anew.

The *Bouvia* case suggests the limit of what patients can ask of health services organizations. At least in California, the law limits what the organization and its managers can do, and the obligation to obey the law guarantees a minimum level of performance. The ethics reflected in the organization's philosophy determine the extent to which it has a higher standard. The law is different in New York (and in cases recently decided in New Jersey), and these differences can only reinforce the need for the organization to be aware of its state's laws and, more importantly, to address these issues prospectively.

NONHOSPITAL ORGANIZATIONS

The case of Henrietta Morrow suggests that the problems of death and dying in nonhospital health services organizations are very similar to those of hospitals. An increasingly aged population and the prospect of AIDS as a chronic, rather than acute, medical problem are two important reasons why nursing facilities (NFs), hospices, and home health agencies should prospectively address the issues raised by death and dying. This means a review from organizational philosophy down to operational policies. The philosophy and policies regarding matters such as life-continuation decisions and artificial hydration and nutrition should be communicated to patients and potential patients and their families.

Somebody Changed the Rules of the Game!

In 1986, Ruth Mittlemann was admitted to the Hebrew Home, a nursing facility. Mittlemann suffered from amyotrophic lateral sclerosis, or Lou Gehrig's disease. Her condition deteriorated gradually, and by late 1989 it was clear that she would soon be unable to swallow, and thus be unable to take food and water by mouth. Before entering the facility, Mittlemann had executed a living will that expressly stated that she did not want to receive artificial hydration or nutrition, and that she wished only to be kept comfortable and be treated for pain once she could no longer swallow. At the time Mittlemann entered the Hebrew Home, her living will posed no problem, because the facility had no organizational policy on this issue.

In early 1988, the board of trustees of the Hebrew Home began work on a policy regarding artificial nutrition and hydration. It was the most rancorous issue that the board had ever considered. Several members resigned because of the intense debate, which sometimes degenerated into personal attacks.

The final result was a policy adopted in late 1988. It stated that the sanctity of life had to be respected, and that only if death were imminent could patients or their surrogates direct that such basic human care as food and water be stopped.

Mittlemann learned of this new policy only when she was told that it would be necessary to place a nasogastric tube so that she could be hydrated and fed. She protested vehemently, and reaffirmed what she had written in her living will. There were other nursing facilities in the area, but Mittlemann liked where she was. She only objected to being forced to receive treatment that she didn't want.

On its face, this change is fundamentally unfair to Mittlemann. She is caught in a problem that is beyond her control and not of her own making. The organization, too, is in an awkward situation. Should it accede to her wishes it violates its now stated philosophy about the sanctity of life.

The principle of respect for persons—specifically, the element of fidelity—should govern here. The organization is obliged to apprise patients of policies that affect them. Since the Hebrew Home had not developed a policy on artificial hydration and nutrition when Mittlemann was first admitted, the trust she had placed in the organization when she chose it would be violated. Offering to move her to another facility does not eliminate the Hebrew Home's duty. As distasteful as it might be to the organization and its board, this case describes a situation that should be treated as an exception to the stated policy.

In 1990, 54-year-old Janet Adkins, who suffered from Alzheimer's disease, sought and received the help of a physician who had developed a device that allows a lethal dose of chemicals to be self-administered. Adkins feared losing her memory and the ability to engage in her normal activities, and she wanted to commit suicide before her mental abilities deteriorated to the point where she could no longer make a rational decision.[39] Commentators have criticized the action and the help given her by the physician as procedurally flawed, and called her competence into question because she had Alzheimer's.[40] This case has brought to the public's attention anew the whole issue of active euthanasia and the right to commit suicide and to be assisted by someone.

The law regarding the criminality of aiding and abetting suicide will have to change before a case such as that of Janet Adkins has implications for health services managers. It is possible, however, that like abortion, suicide will be defined by courts or legislatures as a privacy issue. If so, health services organizations and their managers will have to grapple with the ethical implications of assisted suicide within the context of the organizational philosophy.

CONCLUSION

Ethical problems of death and dying are among the most common the health services organization and its clinical and managerial staff encounter. These issues are often especially difficult because they arise at the beginning and end of life. Technology is central to the ethical and legal problems about death and dying that have arisen recently. New technology may solve some problems, but if history is a guide, technology is as likely to create other dilemmas as it is to solve existing problems. For treatments such as tube feedings, which extend life but are not technology based, the issue is more basic. Food and water are fundamental parts of human existence, and it is difficult to conclude that they represent extraordinary treatment, except under very special circumstances.

Continued attention to the implications of technology for patient autonomy and the principle of nonmaleficence are necessary if the organization is to fulfill its mission within the context of its philosophy. This is a major role of managers, who act as moral agents at the same time that they function as employees of the organization.

NOTES

1. "A Definition of Irreversible Coma," Report of the Harvard Medical School Ad Hoc Committee to Examine the Definition of Brain Death, *Journal of the American Medical Association 205*, no. 6 (August 1968): 337–338.

2. Robert M. Veatch, "Brain Death: Welcome Definition . . . or Dangerous Judgment?" *Hastings Center Report 2*, no. 6 (November 1972): 10.

3. President's Commission for the Study of Ethical Problems in Medicine and Biomedical and Behavioral Research, *Defining Death: Medical, Legal and Ethical Issues in the Determination of Death* (Washington, DC: Government Printing Office, 1981), 25.

4. Personal communication from the Uniform Law Commissioners, Chicago, Illinois, July 26, 1990.

5. Alexander Morgan Capron, "The Report of the President's Commission on the Uniform Determination of Death Act." In *Death: Beyond Whole-Brain Criteria,* edited by Richard M. Zaner (Boston: Kluwer Academic Publishers, 1988), 163.

6. The American Academy of Neurology adopted the National Conference of Commissioners on Uniform State Laws' definition on August 3, 1978. That definition states that "for legal and medical purposes an individual with irreversible cessation of all function of the brain, including the brain stem, is dead. Determination of death under this act shall be made in accordance with reasonable medical standards." (Private communication from the American Academy of Neurology, May 15, 1990.)

7. *In re Quinlan,* 70 N.J. 10, 355 A.2d 647 (1976).

8. Department of Health and Human Services, Office of Human Development Services, Final Rule, Child Abuse and Neglect Prevention and Treatment Program, 45 CFR Part 1340, April 15, 1985.

9. Ibid.

10. Ibid.

11. Editorial, *Hospitals 58,* no. 24 (December 1984): 10.

12. Adapted from Robert M. Veatch, *Case Studies in Medical Ethics* (Cambridge: Harvard University Press, 1977), 340–341. Used with permission.

13. "Significant Gains in Legislation Mark Year at Midpoint," *Newsletter of Concern for Dying and the Society for the Right to Die* (Summer 1990): 2.

14. *"State Health Notes,"* Intergovernmental Health Policy Project, The George Washington University, Washington, DC, No. 33, February 1983, 3.

15. "Medical Durable Power of Attorney," Society for the Right to Die, June 14, 1990.

16. Andrew L. Evans and Baruch A. Brody, "The Do-Not-Resuscitate Order in Teaching Hospitals," *Journal of the American Medical Association 253,* no. 15 (April 1985): 2236–2239.

17. Susanna E. Bedell and Thomas L. Delbanco, "Choices About Cardiopulmonary Resuscitation in the Hospital: When Do Physicians Talk with Patients?" *New England Journal of Medicine 320,* no. 17 (April 1984): 1089–1093.

18. Robert M. Wachter, John M. Luce, Norman Hearst, and Bernard Lo, "Decisions about Resuscitation: Inequities among Patients with Different Diseases but Similar Prognoses," *Annals of Internal Medicine 111,* no. 6 (September 1989): 525–532.

19. Susan Morse, "Final Requests: Preparing for Death," *Washington Post,* July 15, 1985.

20. "Rights and Responsibilities: A National Survey of Healthcare Opinions." Report sponsored by the American Board of Family Practice and conducted by Research and Forecasts, Inc., 1985, 9.

21. S. Van McCrary and Jeffrey R. Botkin, "Hospital Policy on Advance Directives: Do Institutions Ask Patients About Living Wills? *Journal of the American Medical Association 262,* no. 17 (November 1989): 2411–2414.

22. Gerald Kelly, "The Duty to Preserve Life," *Theological Studies 12* (December 1951): 550.

23. "Declaration on Euthanasia," Vatican Congregation for the Doctrine of the Faith, June 26, 1980.

24. Tom L. Beauchamp and James F. Childress, *Principles of Biomedical Ethics,* 3rd ed. (New York: Oxford University Press, 1989), 128.

25. Jay Matthews, "Judge Rejects Palsy Victim's Bid to Starve," *Washington Post,* December 17, 1983.

26. "California Supreme Court Rejects Appeal by Bouvia to Starve," *Washington Post,* January 20, 1984.

27. "Patient Repeatedly Calls Off Her Effort to Starve to Death," *New York Times,* April 24, 1985.

28. "The Latest Word," *Hasting Center Report 15,* no. 4 (August 1985): 36.

29. "Doctors Stop Force-Feeding of Quadraplegic Who Sued," *Washington Post,* April 18, 1986.

30. "Bouvia Moves to Another CA Hospital," *Hospital Week,* American Hospital Association, May 30, 1986.

31. "Right to Refuse Forced Feeding Upheld in Court," *Washington Post,* June 6, 1986.

32. Tinker Ready, "Medical Groups Back Plaintiffs in Right-to-Die Case," *Healthweek,* December 18, 1989.

33. "Patient's Right to Starve Upheld," *Washington Post,* February 3, 1984.

34. Susan M. Wolf, "Nancy Beth Cruzan: In No Voice At All," *Hastings Center Report 20,* no. 1 (January–February 1990): 39.

35. *Cruzan v. Director, Missouri Department of Health et al.* 110 S.Ct.2841.

36. Malcolm Gladwell, "Woman in Right to Die Case Succumbs," *Washington Post,* December 27, 1990.

37. Joanne Lynn and James F. Childress, "Must Patients Always be Given Food and Water?" *Hastings Center Report 13,* no. 5 (October 1983): 17–21; John J. Paris and Anne B. Fletcher, "Infant Doe Regulations and the Absolute Requirements to Use Nourishment and Fluids for the Dying Infant," *Law, Medicine & Health Care 11* (October 1983): 210–213.

38. American Hospital Association, "Withholding and Withdrawing Life-Prolonging Medical Treatment," Press Release, March 15, 1986.

39. Victor Cohn, "An Assisted Suicide: Is It the First Step Toward Euthanasia?" *Washington Post,* Health Section, June 12, 1990.

40. Nancy Gibbs, "Dr. Death's Suicide Machine," *Time,* June 18, 1990.

11

∞

EXPERIMENTATION AND ABORTION

FEW HEALTH SERVICES ORGANIZATIONS perform true clinical experimentation in the form of clinical trials for drugs, biologicals, and devices. Where such research is performed, patients who participate will almost certainly be protected by specific federal requirements, professional guidelines, and internationally recognized codes on experimentation. (Several of these codes are reproduced in Appendix C.) The concept of experimentation includes much more than formal research protocols and clinical trials, however. Under this wider definition, nonstandard diagnostic and therapeutic activities are also experimenting. Both formal and other types of experimentation require more than standard review and consent procedures, for example. Some types of experimentation are unregulated; here, it is up to the organization, through its managers, to protect patients.

The Supreme Court decision in *Roe v. Wade* in 1973 decriminalized abortion by recognizing a constitutionally protected right to abortion in the first trimester, with state limitations permitted only after the first trimester. The result was the rapid development of specialized clinics to perform abortion. Hospitals and other health services organizations looked to their philosophies and underlying moral values to determine whether they should offer such services. The issue of abortion has not yet been resolved. Those opposed to abortion are using political means to overturn *Roe v. Wade*. In the meantime, technology has greatly changed what can be done for the neonate and the abortus. These technological changes will further test the moral philosophies and activities of health services organizations and their managers.

EXPERIMENTATION

Health services managers are likely to think of research and experimentation as exclusive to the academic medical center, where rigorous protection and standards of review are applied. But new uses of existing treatments, drugs, and devices also represent experimenting. "Innovative treatment" is treatment that is neither standard nor experimental, and requires more than normal review and consent procedures. Innovation is a gray and unregulated area. Organizations that use innovative treatment must ensure that their patients are protected. The problem of research is further complicated because, except for some safeguards imposed by state law and voluntary safeguards imposed by the organization itself, surgical experimentation and development of new surgical techniques are uncontrolled. This major gap makes experimentation and innovative therapy of vital concern to the organization and its managers.

No generally recognized ethical codes applied to research until after World War II. Even today, with few exceptions, codes serve only as nonbinding guidelines. Federal regulations that govern certain research are the notable exception.

In 1949, the Nuremberg Military Tribunal identified basic principles of acceptable medical research—later called the Nuremberg Code—when it rendered its opinion following the trial of Nazi physicians who had conducted experiments on prisoners of war and prisoners in concentration camps. Since then, and concomitant with increasing research involving human subjects, several codes and sets of guidelines have been issued. Some, such as the Declaration of Helsinki, are international in scope; others, such as the American Medical Association's (AMA's) Ethical Guidelines for Clinical Investigation and Fetal Research Guidelines and the Department of Health and Human Service's (HHS's) Policy for Protection of Human Research Subjects, are directed toward U.S. practice and activity. These policy statements are presented in Appendix C.

Evidence of the growing attention paid to research was shown in 1974 when Congress established the National Commission for the Protection of Human Subjects of Biomedical and Behavioral Research. The Commission was to identify the basic ethical principles that should underlie research involving human subjects, guidelines for the protection of whom it had a mandate to develop. Emphasis was placed on the unique needs of children, prisoners, and institutionalized people with mental disabilities. The final report focused on the principles of respect for persons, beneficence, and justice, and the National Commission found application for them in informed consent, assessment of risks and benefits, and selection of research subjects.[1] The Commission included the duty not to harm (nonmaleficence) in beneficence; thus, its ethical principles are like those in Chapter 1.

Ethical issues raised by research include the morality of therapeutic versus nontherapeutic experimentation; the need for competent, voluntary, and informed consent; and the morality of experimenting on incompetent subjects, such as people with mental or physical disabilities, and children. Obtaining consent for research is a major problem, as shown by a study of a clinical trial in a teaching hospital that found that 39% of patients, all of whom had supposedly given informed consent and signed consent forms, were not aware that research was involved in induction of their labor.[2] The Nuremberg Code prohibits research on subjects who lack the legal capacity to grant consent—a prohibition that is broad enough to preclude research on children. Other codes, including federal regulations, permit legal guardians to consent to research performed on their children or wards. The unclear definition of innovation, compared with experimentation, causes difficulties in operational settings and in developing adequate consent procedures. The discussion on consent in Chapter 9 is applicable to the ethical problems of research.

It is not easy for hospitals, most of which have no ongoing research programs, to define experimentation and innovative therapy. Nonetheless, definitions are important, not only because they determine whether there is a need to meet legal requirements or form an institutional review board (IRB), but also because the organization must ensure that its own, presumably more rigorous procedures for consent and protecting the patient, are followed. A case example illustrates the problem.

This is Experimenting!?

An internal auditor performed a study of supplies used in biopsies. The data for kidney biopsies revealed major discrepancies: use of biopsy packs exceeded the number of procedures by 50%. The auditor was puzzled, but double checking requisitions and utilization data showed them to be correct. Theft was unlikely.

The auditor made informal inquiries and spoke to technicians in the cytology lab. One agreed to speak confidentially about the additional kidney biopsies. The technician told him a nephrology fellow was using a second pack to take additional tissue during kidney biopsies. The tissue was sent to cytology for special studies ordered by the fellow. The technician said the fellow had a new theory about treating end-stage renal disease.

Is this research? Taking additional tissue or using part of the specimen in the manner described is part of an experiment, even though the act of obtaining it is not itself experimental. By trying to prove or disprove a theory, the nephrology fellow is performing research. Even if the patient had given consent for the initial biopsy, no consent was granted to use the tissue in the manner described. Taking more tissue or a second biopsy puts the patient at additional risk with no actual or potential diagnostic or therapeutic benefit. The organization and its managers have an absolute duty to prevent unauthorized research and policies, and procedures regarding such research should be established. There must also be close monitoring of innovative treatment and, here, the level of concern increases with the degree of risk. Adequacy of consent is critical for both experimentation and innovative therapy.

The case also has an economic dimension. The action by the nephrology fellow adds to the laboratory workload. If these charges (or costs) are paid by third-party payors because they believe they represent part of a patient's diagnosis or treatment, the organization is acting dishonestly toward the payor.

Organizational policies must distinguish unauthorized from authorized experimentation. Extracting a few extra milliliters of amniotic fluid on amniocentesis causes moderate additional risk. Taking unused urine routinely collected for other purposes, or performing analyses on the placenta, poses no risk to the patient, but requires consent nonetheless. Minor risks do not justify ignoring patients' rights and the duties owed them. HHS regulations recognize minimal research risk and permit special review procedures.

Guidelines and Codes

HHS regulations are specific, but affect only HHS-funded research. The Food and Drug Administration (FDA) regulates interstate sale of drugs, biologicals, and devices. This includes new product development, an activity necessarily involving research. FDA regulates neither innovative treatment nor surgical experimentation. Thus, whether coronary artery bypass surgery is sufficiently developed to proceed, or whether radial keratotomy (ophthalmic surgery) can be safely attempted are matters for professional review, scrutiny by the organization, and, in the final analysis, patient recourse through medical malpractice litigation. No national public regulatory review occurs.

Unlike HHS, FDA pays no attention to funding source. FDA is concerned with whether the drug, biological, or device being tested is subject to its authority. If so, FDA will approve a product for sale only if its regulations have been followed during testing. In terms of state laws, only New York state has a general statute regulating research. A few other states, such as Virginia and Wisconsin, regulate research in public and private mental health facilities.

Beyond these governmentally imposed controls, all research is subject only to voluntary ethical guidelines. This means that the human subject must trust the ethical conduct of the researcher (who may also be the caregiver) and the organization through its managers. In these situations, the AMA guidelines on clinical investigation and fetal research are helpful, but must be specifically adapted for each organization. (See Appendix C.)

Several of the ethical issues involved in research were raised in the mid-nineteenth century by an American physician, Dr. William Beaumont, and a French physiologist, Claude Bernard. For 2 years, Beaumont experimented on a man named Alexis St. Martin, who had been injured in the abdomen by a shotgun blast. The wound did not heal properly and St. Martin declined to undergo surgery. The resulting gastric fistula permitted Beaumont to observe the physiology of the stomach.[3] His work with St. Martin prompted Beaumont to formulate a personal ethic in 1833 regarding experimentation that remains relevant today: 1) at times there is no alternative to human experimentation, 2) the experimenter must be conscientious and responsible, 3) random studies are unacceptable, 4) the experiment must be discontinued when it causes distress to the subject, and 5) the experiment must be abandoned at the subject's request.

Claude Bernard, born in 1813, became an eminent physiologist. He wrote about use of live animals in medical research (vivisection), and distinguished the unacceptable from the acceptable by asking whether the purpose of the activity was to mutilate or to learn. He argued that the purpose determines the ethics: if the purpose is to learn, the research is acceptable. He provided a theoretical basis for the ethics of human experimentation:

> Physicians make therapeutic experiments daily on their patients, and surgeons perform vivisections daily on their subjects. Experiments, then, may be performed on man, but within what limits? It is our duty and our right to perform an experiment on man whenever it can save his life, cure him, or gain him some personal benefit. The principle of medical and surgical morality, therefore consists in never performing on man an experiment which might be harmful to him to any extent, even though the result might be highly advantageous to science, i.e., to the health of others. But performing experiments and operations exclusively from the point of view of the patient's own advantage does not prevent their turning out profitably to science.[4]

Bernard's guidelines stress therapeutic research (i.e., experimental treatments applied in an effort to benefit the patient). (The distinction between therapeutic and nontherapeutic is discussed later in this section.)

In the sense that research is defined as attempting new means, methods, and techniques, the medical community has always performed research. Without innovation, medical knowledge would have stagnated. If medicine is to continue to progress, experimentation and innovative treatment must be continued. Protecting the human subject remains difficult and problematic, however.

Fever All through the Night

Assistant Administrator Beverley Atchison finished reading the minutes of the utilization review committee. Atchison noted that a lengthy discussion had occurred with regard to the seemingly overlong stay of a pediatric case. In fact, the attending pediatrician had appeared before the committee to explain the length of stay and the unique regimen of treatment.

The case involved a child who developed a fever of unknown etiology. The child was hospitalized and routine tests showed no pathology. The physician explained that she had read about fever therapy in the literature and was impressed with the possibilities it offered. Therefore, she decided to determine its appropriateness in cases of fever with unknown etiology. She ordered Tylenol if the fever went above 102.5°. Otherwise, there was to be no intervention.

The pediatrician stated that her treatment proved itself, because after 3 days the child had an uneventful recovery. However, the therapy raised numerous questions among the committee members.

This treatment regimen is innovative; it might even be classified as experimental. The case raises two issues. Did the child's parents receive adequate information about the therapy to give informed consent? This question bears directly on how the hospital determines whether informed consent is obtained in cases such as these. Since the therapy was innovative, special approval and procedures should have been used.

If this therapy does qualify as experimental rather than innovative, the second issue is the important distinction of whether it was therapeutic or nontherapeutic research. Experimental treatment that might benefit the subject is therapeutic—the subject is also the patient. Nontherapeutic research involves healthy subjects, or patients with medical problems other than those at which the experimental treatment is directed. Closer attention should be given to nontherapeutic research because the subject will not benefit from the research. Special emphasis should be put on the quality of consent. Some commentators believe that nontherapeutic and nondiagnostic research on children and on adults who are legally incompetent, should be prohibited.[5]

Notable in the case is the nursing staff's lack of attention to the unusual orders for this child's care. Nursing's code of ethics emphasizes protecting the patient, and requires the nurse to intervene if the patient is unnecessarily at risk. Timely reporting should have been made through the nursing hierarchy.

All codes emphasize the subject's voluntary and informed consent. Competence is given less attention. The Nuremberg Code (1949) includes a provision stating that subjects should be able to halt the experiment when they no longer wish to continue. But this places a potentially impossible burden on the subject, who may become incapacitated by the experiment itself or by an unrelated medical problem, or may be intimidated by the setting or the personalities involved. Subjects are also likely to lack the technical competence to know when their safety is threatened. This weakness was partially corrected in the Declaration of Helsinki (1964, revised 1975), which recommended establishing an independent committee to review and approve the experimental protocol. This committee is required by HHS. (The role, composition, and function of the IRB were discussed in Chapter 5.)

All codes and guidelines permit nontherapeutic research. They recognize that volunteers for whom the experimental treatment offers no diagnostic or therapeutic advantage are needed for certain types of research. There is clear utilitarian language in all codes (except the AMA guidelines, which have a strong element of paternalism), which compares and balances risk to the subject (in the case of nontherapeutic research) with the benefit to society. Conversely, the emphasis on voluntary and informed consent suggests a Kantian philosophy, and is reflected in the principles of respect for persons and non-maleficence. This view is also found in HHS regulations.

A major difficulty with research codes other than federal regulations is that they inadequately separate the physician's roles as healer and researcher. This combination places a heavy ethical burden on the physician because the duality of interests puts the physician-researcher in a classic conflict of interest situation. What is good for the research subject as a patient is not necessarily good for the experimental design. This problem is exacerbated when nontherapeutic research is undertaken, because then the risk to the subject is not balanced by potential benefit. AMA guidelines recognize the dilemma, but adopt a paternalistic view of the relationship between physician and patient-subject. The physician is expected to exercise professional skill and judgment to act in the patient's best interests.

Falsification of Research Data

A unique twist to problems in research occurred in the late 1970s and early 1980s.[6] John Darsee, a fellow in cardiology at Emory University and Harvard University and a brilliant physician of unusual talent, perpetrated an amazing fraud. Darsee was found to have falsified large quantities of research data on the genetic and biochemical factors affecting heart disease. Some of these data had been used in publications in leading medical journals. Other data were being used for papers in process. Many of the articles listed prominent physician-researchers in the field as coauthors; however, some later asserted they were unaware they were listed as coauthors.

Darsee's champions supported him until evidence of his deception proved overwhelming. Darsee's detractors argued that his supporters were too easily charmed by his personality and talents. When researchers and administrators at Emory and Harvard learned of the fraud, they withdrew papers and abstracts that had been submitted for publication. The only step that could be taken regarding articles that had already been published was to urge potential users to disregard them. It is claimed that no patients were harmed because of Darsee's clinical work. While this is verifiable by review of records at the hospitals involved, much more potential harm lies in the fact that Darsee's publication list includes over 100 articles and abstracts. There is no way for readers unaware of the fraud to know which of them contain false data.

The organizations involved acted forthrightly when the problems were uncovered. What happened violated both research ethics and proscriptions imposed by funding organizations, such as the National Institutes of Health. The real questions, however, are those concerning the adequacy of surveillance, not only of Darsee, but of all physicians in training who engage in research and collect research data. Subsequent self-assessment at Emory led to new safeguards to review the work of physicians in training and to monitor the use of names of teaching staff as authors on publications by residents. Research findings are also reviewed much more extensively since the Darsee affair. With all these protections, it is still conceded that "(it) won't prevent the generation of fraudulent data, but under this system someone like Darsee couldn't send out articles at the rate of one a week without raising suspicions."[7]

Summary

Regulations such as those of HHS focus responsibility on the organization and members of the IRB. Irrespective of legal requirements, the organization and its managers have an ethical responsibility and independent duties under the principles of respect for persons, beneficence, nomalficence, and even justice (e.g., equitable selection of research subjects) to protect and serve the patient. Managers must put in place the systems and procedures to prevent unauthorized research, and to provide the necessary extra protection when innovative treatment is proposed or undertaken. The Darsee affair raises a whole new set of potential problems in teaching and research institutions. The most important element is awareness on the part of all staff about the parameters of acceptable practice and their willingness to act or speak out, when necessary.

ABORTION

Few issues in biomedical ethics have sparked such raging controversy as abortion. In 1973, the U.S. Supreme Court handed down opinions in the *Roe v. Wade* and *Doe v. Bolton* cases that prohibited states from interfering with a woman's right to have an abortion during the first trimester of pregnancy, and that limited state interference in the second and third trimesters.[8] The Court established 28 weeks as the lower limit of fetal viability. This limit is increasingly being challenged by improved technology that can keep premature infants alive and allow them to mature. A study using 1986–1988 data found that neonatal survival to 30 days ranged from 20% at 24 weeks to 94% at 29 weeks.[9] The authors concluded that their findings represent a significant increase in survival and a decrease in early morbidity compared with studies of similar populations performed before 1986. Efforts to make significant improvements in survival rates of neonates below 24 weeks must await improved technology.

The Court's reasoning was based on a right to privacy, which it found implicit in the Constitution. The decision legalizing abortion marked a major change in American political and social life. Previously, the widespread illegality of abortion had determined policy for most health services organizations; now, for the first time, they had to consider the morality of abortion.

Abortion is an emotionally charged issue, and the debate on it has tended to generate more heat than light. It is an especially difficult problem—there is scant middle ground, and thus little room for compromise. Underlying the abortion issue is women's desire to achieve reproductive equality. Pro-choice arguments are based on respect for privacy and the right of women to determine their own destinies, including the use of their bodies. Pro-life advocates argue that human life is at stake, and that the concept of personhood adopted by the Supreme Court took no account of the fact that the fetus develops into an infant, who is entitled to the protections offered by the Constitution. More recent Supreme Court decisions (e.g, *Webster v. Reproductive Health Services*) have upheld state legislation that applies a variety of protections to the fetus and limitations on abortion services.[10] The abortion debate suggests the complexity of the relationship between ethics and law. Even though abortion is legal, the right to have an abortion is challenged by those who do not consider it morally right.

Following the Supreme Court's decision legalizing abortion, large numbers of clinics and counseling centers were established to meet the sudden new demand for abortions. Many hospitals viewed performing abortions as simply another lawful medical service consistent with their organizational philosophy to serve the community. Some sectarian hospitals also found the decision simple: for them, abortion was killing a human being and was immoral. Nonsectarian organizations may have come to the same conclusion, perhaps for different reasons.

Courts have generally permitted private (nongovernmental) hospitals to exercise their organizational philosophy without interference. This means they can refuse to perform abortions or other procedures that they find morally repugnant. Some states have prohibited publicly funded hospitals from performing abortions—a change from the past, when public hospitals were expected to perform all legal procedures. Virtually all states have statutes with "conscience" clause provisions that permit private organizations and their staffs to refuse to perform abortions or sterilizations. Congress has passed a similar law that affects legislation that authorizes federal programs. It prohibits public authorities and officials from imposing requirements that are contrary to religious beliefs or moral convictions (e.g., abortions or sterlizations). Regardless of conscience clauses, organizations must be cognizant of the need to accommodate staff members whose moral beliefs do not allow them to participate in such procedures. A common sense response has been to excuse persons who object to abortions and sterilizations from participating in such procedures. This may not eliminate the discontinuities and conflict such ethical issues can cause in an organization, however.

The concept of personhood enunciated in *Roe* and *Bolton* represents a legal determination that birth confers major changes in legal status. At birth, the infant becomes a person, and is entitled to constitutional protections. As noted above, however, states have increasingly enacted legislation to protect the fetus. To those who see abortion as a moral question, legal determinations are insufficient. Few differences distinguish the neonate from the late-term fetus. The neonate is as dependent on adults as is the fetus, although for neonates the mother need not be the exclusive provider of sustenance and protection. The Supreme Court's view about first, second, and third trimester abortions, as evidenced in cases subsequent to *Roe* and *Bolton,* squares with a commonly held belief that early abortions are morally more acceptable than those performed later in the term. This logic requires that everything else equal, the more mature the fetus, the greater must be impediments to abortion.

Why Bother?

Dr. Stangardd is a neonatologist at State University Hospital. He recently completed his residency and was hired to join the three other neonatologists on staff. Previously, he practiced at a facility that did not perform abortions. Thus, although he had read about the problem of what treatment should be given viable premature fetuses produced after abortion, he had not witnessed such a case.

Stangardd was having lunch in the cafeteria when his beeper sounded. He called the unit and was told that a late-term fetus resulting from an abortion had just been brought there from the OR. The nurse on the phone told him that his boss, the chief of neonatology, wanted him in the unit immediately. Stangardd spoke, half to himself, as he ran toward the neonatal unit, "How silly! On one floor they're trying to destroy the fetus, and on another they're trying to save the product of that abortion. Somebody ought to resolve this incredible contradiction."

This hospital faces a moral dilemma. Had this case occurred in California after 1976, the hospital would have had to take "all reasonable steps, except extraordinary means, in accordance with good medical practice, to preserve the life and health of the live-born person."[11] Subsequently, other states enacted laws with similar provisions.

Federal Law

Congressional enactment has superseded California law. It does not resolve the moral paradox Dr. Stangardd noted, however. As discussed in Chapter 10, The Child Abuse Amendments of 1984 (P.L. 98-457) limit the choices available regarding treating infants with life-threatening medical problems. The regulations define infancy as beginning at live birth, regardless of the circumstances of that birth. With or without the law, however, State University Hospital is trying to meet the woman's constitutional right to have an abortion. At the same time, it seeks to fulfill a humanitarian philosophy to save life—even that of an unwanted fetus. The dilemma of legitimate, competing claims will become even starker as neonatology is able to save premature infants at earlier gestational ages. In terms of resource allocation under the principle of justice, clinicians fail in their duty to use resources efficiently if they apply heroic measures to live premature fetuses with no hope of survival when neither federal law nor the concept of extraordinary care requires it.

One aspect of abortion adds a dimension of considerable complexity: experimentation. What safeguards should apply to experimenting on a fetus that is about to be aborted and that will certainly not survive the procedure? To whom does the fetus belong? Who may consent to the experiment? May nontherapeutic experimentation be done on a liveborn fetus that cannot be saved (nonviable)? HHS guidelines answer questions like these by protecting the fetus through limitations on nontherapeutic experimentation whether *in utero* or *ex utero,* and by requiring parental consent. HHS regulations apply only to programs funded by HHS. Activities on and disposition of dead fetuses are regulated by the states.

Logic might suggest that if a fetus *in utero* is not entitled to protection of the law in terms of its continued existence, experimentation can be done without limitation. HHS does not take this position. Of course, after live birth the mantle of personhood is conferred upon the fetus *qua* infant, and it has legal protections. Fetal experimentation raises many questions, and they are among the most difficult in biomedical ethics. Resolving them will surely test the organization's philosophy and the manager's personal ethic. To fail to work toward that end, however, does a disservice to all involved, including the liveborn fetus and the fetus *in utero.*

In 1989, HHS stopped funding fetal research, thus effectively ending it in the United States. The long-term implications of this decision for the medical promise held by the results of fetal experimentation are uncertain.

A particularly poignant and compelling case that seems to justify an abortion occurred in California, where a brain-diseased woman had great difficulty obtaining an abortion for a 21-week fetus she was carrying. Most facilities contacted on her behalf considered the physical risk too high. The woman suffered from a nervous system disorder known as Huntington's chorea, a rare hereditary disease that causes mental deterioration and involuntary movements. She was physically incapacitated and totally incoherent. She had spent more than 3 years in restraints in nursing homes. Her pregnancy resulted from a rape that occurred during institutionalization. Her disorder made it unlikely that she was even aware of what happened to her.[12]

Denying an abortion on clinical grounds is always morally justified and would be required under the principle of nonmaleficence. If a health services organization is to provide an abortion only on substantive grounds, this case provides some of the most compelling facts imaginable. An organizational philosophy with an absolute prohibition could make no exception.

There is little middle ground in the debate over abortion. Nonetheless, progress toward a compromise might begin with the premise that fetal life should not be ended easily. It can be terminated only after applying standards of due process and substantial cause. A starting point is the premise that some reasons for an abortion carry more weight than others. To many, termination of pregnancies resulting from rape or incest, significant genetic anomalies, and major risk to the mother's health are morally more justifiable than pregnancies terminated because of the sex of the fetus or because of social convenience. Once reasons for abortion are distinguished, criteria can be developed to consider the appropriateness (morality) of abortions. Such an approach limits the pro-choice position to have abortion legal and freely available; it also limits the pro-life position that no fetus may be killed. It is in such middle ground that constructive debate could occur.

Summary

Technologically, more problems—but also more answers—lie ahead. Infants can be saved at earlier gestational ages. Although advances in neonatology are a boon to premature infants, they cause ethical problems about resource allocation in cost-conscious hospitals. The other horn of the dilemma is the federal requirement that medically indicated care cannot be denied to infants with disabilities who have life-threatening conditions except when the treating physician determines that certain conditions are present. These conditions were noted in Chapter 10. A liveborn product of abortion meets this definition, thus complicating the issue of abortion.

A partial answer to the morality of abortion for pro-life advocates may lie with techniques that permit an unwanted fetus to be extracted undamaged and implanted in a surrogate mother, or even in an artificial womb. This does not, however, solve the problem of what to do if the woman does not want her child to survive. The question remains, too, of who pays for the care of an unwanted fetus, and this raises the issue of justice in resource allocation. One answer is that prospective adoptive parents should pay the costs of bringing the fetus to term. A precedent has been set by surrogate mothers, whose medical expenses and economic losses during pregnancy are covered by the adoptive parents.

CONCLUSION

A great deal of research on new drugs is now done outside the United States, especially in Third World countries. Applications for new drugs have declined in the United States. It is alleged that rigorous federal controls in the past 2 decades have caused these changes. Those who put greater weight on the social utility of medical progress urge that requirements for experimentation be made less onerous. At the same time, however, enhanced protections have been demanded for those groups with diminished autonomy, such as military personnel and prisoners. The inherently dynamic nature of research means that more changes lie ahead.

Research suggests that much has to be done to protect patient autonomy, as well as to involve patients in consent processes during experimentation. The majority of the burden in this regard lies with the physician, who is qualified to describe the risks and benefits of innovative therapy and therapeutic experimentation, or the risks of nontherapeutic experimentation. Nonetheless, the manager remains a critical component in the equation, and is a moral agent who acts to perfect the patient's rights.

Abortion continues to be a major societal issue. By now, sufficient time has elapsed so that health services organizations and their managers have resolved the issue internally. It is in this process that the organization's philosophy and mission play a critical role. Two recent developments may affect the equilibrium. First, pro-life groups are determined to bring about change in the legal status of abortion. Second, technology available through *in utero* surgery and neonatal intensive care units permits physicians to save fetuses earlier and earlier. Developments like these will cause reappraisal of the issues. Managers must be prepared to address their ethical implications.

NOTES

1. The National Commission was established by the National Research Service Award Act of 1974, Public Law 93-348. Its final report was entitled "Belmont Report: Ethical Principles and Guidelines for the Protection of Human Subjects of Research." (Letter of transmittal and report to the President, National Commission for the Protection of Human Subjects of Biomedical and Behavioral Research, September 30, 1978 [DHEW Publication No. [OS] 78-0012], 1978.) In addition, there are special reports and recommendations for research involving children and prisoners.

2. Bradford H. Gray, *Human Subjects in Medical Experimentation: A Sociological Study of the Conduct and Regulation of Clinical Research* (New York: John Wiley & Sons, 1975), 129.

3. Carl J. Wiggers, "Human Experimentation as Exemplified by the Career of Dr. William Beaumont," *Alumni Bulletin,* Western Reserve School of Medicine, 1950, 60–64.

4. Claude Bernard, *An Introduction to the Study of Experimental Medicine* (U.S.: Henry Schuman, Inc., 1927), 101.

5. Paul Ramsey, "Research Involving Children or Incompetents." In *The Patient as Person* (New Haven: Yale University Press, 1970), 252.

6. *Emory Magazine,* December, 1983, 6–15.

7. Ibid., 15.

8. *Roe v. Wade,* 93 S.Ct. 705 (1973); *Doe v. Bolton,* 93 S.Ct. 739 (1973).

9. Brian Wood, Vern Katz, Carl Bose, Robert Goolsby, and Ernest Kraybill, "Survival and Morbidity of Extremely Premature Infants Based on Obstetric Assessment of Gestational Age," *Obstetrics & Gynecology 74* (December 1989): 889.

10. *Webster v. Reproductive Health Services,* 109 S.Ct. 3040 (1989).

11. Sissela Bok, "The Unwanted Child: Caring for the Fetus Born Alive After An Abortion," *Hastings Center Report 6,* no. 5 (October 1976): 10.

12. Christine Russell, "Invalid Undergoes Perilous Abortion," *Washington Post,* June 26, 1985.

V

∞

EMERGING ETHICAL ISSUES

MORE CHANGES HAVE OCCURRED IN the management of health services organizations since the 1970s than have occurred during the years 1900–1970. Rapid change will continue in the future, perhaps even at an accelerating pace. New managerial challenges will put heavier demands on organizational philosophies and the manager's personal ethic. Managers with an ill-defined personal ethic will feel adrift in a world that will seem to have few solid foundations.

Part V consists of Chapter 12, which examines marketing in a competitive environment, and Chapter 13, which analyzes the impact of acquired immunodeficiency syndrome (AIDS) on health services organizations. Both issues developed recently in the health services field and the ethical implications they raise will require special attention.

The competitive environment has convinced the managers of many health services organizations that marketing is essential to their survival. The function of marketing is not new to most health services managers, but applying it in a more commercial and entrepreneurial manner is, and many managers are uncertain of its implications, especially if they manage not-for-profit organizations.

The last chapter addresses AIDS. This disease and its ethical implications will affect all aspects of the operation of all types of health services organizations. It is a major ethical issue of the 1990s, one that health services managers must be prepared to address.

12

∞

MARKETING IN A
COMPETITIVE ENVIRONMENT
AN ADMINISTRATIVE ISSUE

ALTHOUGH THE ELEMENTS OF MARKETING—product, place, promotion, and pricing—have been applied to health services with apparent ease in recent years, the purposes and the context of health services differ from those of the typical business enterprise.

In the 1920s, President Calvin Coolidge noted that the business of America is business. This premise remains accurate: the United States continues to be a bastion of capitalism. Unique among its businesses, however, is the health services segment. Health services differ from other businesses in terms of purpose, type of service provided, orientation, and motives. Unlike most other businesses, health services providers may be affiliated with a particular religion and may have not-for-profit status. Health services organizations are also unique in that they maintain close ties to several professions and provide services that have emotional and psychological aspects. A health services organization is a social enterprise with an economic dimension, rather than an economic enterprise with a social dimension.

Cunningham has noted that marketing in a traditional business enterprise differs from marketing of health services in that the former uses marketing to create demand for its product and to promote and sell its goods and services aggressively.[1] This distinction is sometimes blurred. All health services organizations market, and they have always done so. This is especially true for acute care hospitals and is increasingly true in managed care and nursing facilities (NFs). Historically, marketing occurred in a variety of ways, including community "health days," and press releases. But the new milieu of the competitive marketplace makes marketing something more.

NEED VERSUS DEMAND

Many individuals and organizations in the health services field differ over whether demand is being created or being met. An important dimension of this issue is disagreement as to which types of health services merit creation of demand and which do not. Few would disagree on the importance of creating consumer demand for screening for hypertension or colorectal cancer. The desirability of such efforts is tempered, however, by considerations of costs and benefits; depending on the population and the disease for which screening is done, screening may be unacceptably expensive when measured by the number of true positives found. Both price and nonprice competition may increase demand, but there is general agreement that competition, in and of itself, is desirable. Despite this acceptance of competition, there is likely to be disagreement as to the appropriateness of demand, depending on the medical conditions being treated. Some conditions that objectively require medical intervention may be treated with more than one type of therapy. Coronary artery bypass surgery for patients with mild or moderate symptoms of heart disease is an example of an expensive therapy with mixed results. Cardiac surgeons note the procedure's usefulness for occluded coronary arteries and the relief of angina. Cardiologists and internists are inclined to treat persons with these diagnoses medically. They rely on data that show similar long-term results for patients in some categories when managed with a medical rather than a surgical regimen. Cost differences are enormous. A National Heart Institute study estimates that about 25,000 of the 200,000 bypass procedures performed each year could be foregone, with a savings of $15,000 – $40,000 per surgery.[2]

Contrasted with the objective need to intervene in the case of coronary artery disease are situations that are more subjective. Cosmetic surgery is often cited as a clear example of an "unnecessary" medical service. It is claimed that face lifts, tummy tucks, and silicone implants waste medical resources (whether or not they are paid for by the patient) and that these resources should be available for other uses. This is a subjective definition of need. Reasonable persons could reach different conclusions, as to what patients "need" and whether the demand that arises from that need should be met by the health care system. Perhaps activities such as cosmetic surgery should not be defined as health services at all, but as consumer services (like haircutting and bodybuilding) that happen to use some parts of the health system.

Epidemiologic studies should be used to develop data about populations. These data reveal the incidence and prevalence of diseases, as well as psychological and physical concerns of the population that may fall outside the more traditional definitions of disease. The real problem in terms of assessing need and demand arises when persons judging such data apply their value systems to determine the problem's importance. These judgments make the process less than objective whether it be in determining what should be studied or what is to be done with the results. In turn, these decisions affect the choice of regimens and decisions to treat or not to treat.

The debate about need becomes most heated when issues of marketing ethics are included, especially if marketing is to be used to affect demand or to encourage persons to seek elective procedures. Physical or psychological conditions about which an individual is either unaware or not prepared to treat represent potential demand for medical services. Conditions for which no help is sought because of financial barriers also represent potential demand. Examples include dental care, hammer toes, hemorrhoids, cataracts, and psychiatric services. Troubling in this debate is any suggestion that meeting potential demand is unethical.

If one applies the admittedly broad World Health Organization definition of health,* all efforts to improve health are beneficial. It is instructive to consider wellness (prevention) activities. The possibilities for involvement by the health services organization are almost limitless because every facet of life could be affected to improve general health and prevent medical problems. In addition to wellness activities there are questions of how to treat demand for services that may seem foolish to some observers. Should people be denied elective procedures such as cosmetic surgery simply because other people judge such procedures as trivial, or because what they seek to correct is not life threatening? This level of infringement on individual autonomy is greater than the public is likely to accept at this point in history.

It is not clear how and by whom need and demand are to be judged. Despite the presence of the occasional hypochondriac or Munchausen's syndrome patient, demand for services should be accepted as rational. In looking at demand for medical services, it is most useful to focus attention on the majority of patients. When that group hears about new medical problems or treatment and diagnostic possibilities, it responds rationally. These are the "worried well"— persons not clinically ill, but concerned about their health.

RESPONSIBLE MARKETING

How does the health services organization market services to patients and potential patients in a fashion consistent with its ethical obligation to avoid creating "unnecessary" demand, while at the same time fulfilling its obligation to seek out and serve those who might be in need?

The American Hospital Association (AHA) has developed a statement on the legitimate purposes of hospital advertising, an important element of marketing. According to the AHA, hospitals should advertise to educate the public about available services, to educate the public about health care, to win public support, to be publicly accountable, and to recruit employees. Advertising must be truthful, accurate and fair. Comparisons with other providers, claims of prominence, and promotion of individual professionals should be avoided.[3]

This kind of marketing is responsible marketing. If profits and return on

---

*"Health is a state of complete physical, mental, and social well-being and not merely the absence of disease or infirmity." John J. Hanlon and George E. Pickett, *Public Health: Administration and Practice* (St. Louis: Times Mirror/Mosby, 1984), p. 5.

investment are the primary reasons corporations exist, corporations will have a much different view of what is responsible marketing, as well as what is appropriate competition. This is the difference between giving people whatever they want and tempering desires and potential demand with some attempt to judge value and usefulness. This view of the patient has elements of paternalism, but it is consistent with the purpose set forth in the organization's mission statement.

Demarketing to Avoid Bankruptcy

Chris Hines had finally gotten down far enough in the stack of papers on her desk to get to last month's emergency department (ED) activity report. She had already digested the grim news about the continued financial hemorrhage affecting Community Hospital. The current deficit was $500,000—and it was only the 4th month of the fiscal year. Because Community Hospital served a largely inner city population, many of whom were uninsured or whose care was paid by a chronically underfunded Medicaid program, there seemed to be little hope of the financial situation improving.

Hines knew that over 40% of Community Hospital's admissions came through the ED, and that about half of those admissions arrived by taxi, by private automobile, or on foot. The other half was brought in by the ambulance service run by the city government. Hines had tried to implement a plan to increase the number of elective admissions (and thus improve the payor mix) by encouraging physicians to bring their patients to Community. This effort failed, however, largely because of the difficulty physicians had in getting their private patients admitted— ED admissions were taking too many beds. Hines then tried to work with city officials to implement a new ambulance routing system that would give Community a chance to improve its financial condition. This effort also failed, as city officials were unsympathetic.

Hines knew that Community Hospital's endowment would carry the hospital about 3 years, but that the hospital would be forced to close if it was not breaking even by then. Since there was nothing that could be done with the city, Hines concluded that the key to survival lay with reducing the number of uninsured and Medicaid admissions through the ED.

Hines spoke with several marketing consultants, one of whom offered to do *pro bono* work for Community Hospital. He seized upon the idea of "demarketing" the ED. He reasoned that it was the fine reputation Community Hospital's ED had in the community that was largely responsible for the 50% of ED patients who came other than by city ambulance. He then set out to identify ways in which the ED could be made less attractive to potential patients. The plan he developed included: reducing

ED staffing to the very minimum, closing the parking lot near the ED, reducing housekeeping services so that the physical plant would be dirty and unkempt, deferring all nonsafety-related maintenance, changing the triage policies, procedures, and staffing so as to increase waiting time for nonemergency patients, using staff who were most likely to be rude and inconsiderate, and encouraging rumors that the closure of the ED was imminent.

The consultant knew there might be repercussions beyond the ED, but Community was desperate, and he believed there was no choice but to take extreme action.

In analyzing this case, one must first ask whether there were not other steps that Hines and her managers could have taken to improve the financial condition of Community Hospital. Examples include: closing the ED rather than demarketing it (this approach seems the more honest); undertaking other, more remunerative, medical care activities to offset the ED losses; or opening less costly primary care clinics to care for the worried well and other nonemergency medical problems who were coming into the ED.

Assuming, however, that such options were unavailable, the demarketing strategy raises ethical issues. First, the steps contemplated are likely negatively to affect the quality of care in the ED. Beyond staffing and the physical aspects that are directly affected, the psychological effects on ED staff (rippling into the inpatient side of the hospital, as well) will negatively affect morale and ultimately the quality of care. This violates the principles of beneficence and nonmaleficence.

A second ethical issue raised is justice. People in the community are caught between the city bureaucracy and the efforts of Community Hospital to remain financially viable. They may have little choice but to go to the ED at Community Hospital and endure the indignities and reduction in quality of care resulting from the demarketing strategy. Deliberately adding insult to injury should give all concerned a great deal of discomfort. Another dimension of justice is the unfairness associated with forcing the remaining ED staff to work under such conditions. They will bear the brunt of angry patients and the delapidated, depressing environment.

The fact that the declining financial condition of Community Hospital might have eventually resulted in many of the same changes in the ED is no justification for deliberately undertaking them in the manner contemplated in the case. Desperate people may commit desperate acts, but this does not justify them morally.

FUTURE OF COMPETITION

There is a theory in political science that suggests that over time enemies begin to take on one another's attributes. This concern deeply troubles the not-for-profit sector of the health services system, which views itself as holding values that differ from those held by the for-profit sector. They fear that as they compete for market share, they will be forced to stress financial considerations and economic survival, thus causing them to lose sight of humanitarian motives.

In this regard, prospective payment systems are especially significant. One type of prospective payment system is diagnosis-related groups (DRGs), the Medicare payment scheme. Its effect on health services delivery is beginning to be noticed. Some writers suggest that pressures of DRG payment will lead to an adversarial relationship between patients and organizations (and perhaps the physician), and that patients' interests will be smothered by the demands of efficiency and economic survival. Such results are possible under any payment system or ownership, and will occur whenever caregivers and managers lose sight of their reason for being. Doing more with less need not be at variance with efforts to operationalize the principles of respect for persons, beneficence, nonmaleficence, and justice. It remains for all who are involved in organizing, planning, and delivering health services to keep these principles firmly in mind.

COMPETITION AND PERSONNEL POLICY

Competition has implications for hiring practices as well.

Hiring the Competition

> The two NFs in town are highly competitive. This has caused them to oppose one another's certificate of need (CON) applications to the point of suing each other. The chief operating officers (COOs) of the NFs have been friends since before they joined their respective NFs. They play golf monthly. The COO of one NF is fired after running afoul of the medical director. The other COO offers to hire him as a consultant.

This situation is not covered by any code of ethics. The fired COO is privy to proprietary information that would give the other NF a competitive advantage. In theory, it is possible that the fired COO could consult on matters that would not require him to reveal proprietary knowledge. Given the history of the two organizations, however, this is unlikely. The ethically superior answer would be not to hire the former competitor. Short of that, it might be possible scrupulously to avoid using the competitor's proprietary information. Whether this would be possible would have to be determined by looking more closely at the details of the case.

Does a fired COO have any remaining duty to a former employer? Managers have an ethical duty to keep proprietary information confidential after they sever relations with their employer. This duty of confidentiality continues until events have overtaken the confidential information. If this were not the case, organizations would be hostage to former employees who seek revenge. Managers would be among the first to agree that this is undesirable, both from a managerial and a professional perspective.

SOCIAL RESPONSIBILITY

Changes in the health services field such as the advent of marketing and competition have raised a number of concerns. Some of them were addressed by the Society for Hospital Planning, when, in a "dear colleague" letter, some members expressed fears about the future of hospital planning. These fears are shown in Table 6. These concerns prompted the authors of the letter to request that the board of directors and membership discuss their implications. Self-analysis and debates such as these are important and should continue, both inside and outside the health services field.

Table 6. Desirable characteristics of hospital competition

Features of hospital planning model as we see it developing within society programs and membership	Desired characteristics of hospital planning guided by sense of community service and social conscience
Encourage a corporate and institutional focus.	Encourage a market area and stakeholder (including consumer) focus.
Beat competitors into failure on a product-line basis and gain greater share of local health care market even, if necessary, at a cost to competitors.	Compete to stimulate other providers to offer better services at more reasonable prices *and* to ensure the availability of comprehensive services and care throughout all market segments (not just the easy full-pay/ self-pay segments).
Collect market share data to monitor progress in out-distancing competitors.	Collect market share data to use in areawide determination of trends in consumer use and preference.
Encourage product-line focus for use of resources and managerial and organizational structure.	Encourage community-based networks of services and product groupings that maximize public access to high-quality service at reasonable prices.
Concentrate on organization and management structure vis-à-vis hospital strategy.	Explicitly address the hospital's "corporate culture and values" as the parameters within which strategy is to be developed and pursued.
Encourage a preoccupation with the bottom line and an emphasis on institutional survival.	Stimulate a rejuvenated debate over the ethics of who has access to care, who pays for care, where care is received, and our commitment to community service and humanitarian goals.

From *Hospital Planning and Marketing,* July–August 1984, published by the American Hospital Association, copyright 1984.

So, too, will the debate continue about social responsibility and service versus profitability. AHA national data show that 4.1% of 1983 gross patient revenues at nongovernmental not-for-profit hospitals went toward uncompensated care. The figure for investor-owned hospitals was 3.1%. Uncompensated care accounted for 11.5% of gross patient revenue at state and local government hospitals.[4] Similar results have been found in a study of California hospitals.[5]

A study by the Institute of Medicine of the National Academy of Sciences presented data from four states in which more than 30% of hospitals are for profit. In Florida, Tennessee, Texas, and Virginia, not-for-profit hospitals provided significantly more uncompensated care than did for-profit hospitals. In these four states, uncompensated care in investor-owned hospitals ranged from 3.4% to 3.8% of gross patient revenues, whereas uncompensated care accounted for 5.5%–9.0% in not-for-profit hospitals. The report acknowledged that:

> Such differences could be caused by factors (the size or location of an institution, for instance) other than willingness or reluctance to turn away uninsured patients untreated. But the majority of the committee agreed that the comparatively low levels of uncompensated care in investor-owned hospitals that constitute 30–40 per cent of the hospitals in a state suggest that the presence of such hospitals lessens access to care among people who lack means to pay, and may exacerbate the difficulties faced by hospitals that serve such patients.[6]

All of these studies were marred by methodological problems; the definitive study remains to be done. It is clear, however, that one must be very cautious in attributing motives and results based solely on ownership. A recent study confirmed that not-for-profit hospitals appear more likely to be accessible to the uninsured and medically indigent than are for-profit hospitals. Moreover, not-for-profit hospitals appear more likely to carry a heavier indigent load, and for-profit hospitals appear to serve relatively more patients with "good" insurance. The same study found, however, that for-profit hospitals appear to be more efficient than not-for-profits.[7] The AHA has not provided data on uncompensated care by for-profit and not-for-profit hospitals since 1983, but it determined that in 1988 hospitals spent $8.3 billion on unsponsored care, which it defined as uncompensated care less state and local tax appropriations.[8]

We've Earned It—We'll Keep It!

Freeland Hospital was located in an affluent neighborhood in a suburban community. It had a Medicare census of less than 20% and it received less than 1% of its revenues from Medicaid. Uncollectibles were below 3%. Freeland Hospital's financial situation was extremely solid.

Sherwood Shurmann had been the chief executive officer (CEO) of Freeland for almost 20 years and was justifiably proud of the changes and improvements that he had achieved during his tenure. One of his achievements had been to establish the

Freeland Hospital Foundation, Inc., which received charitable donations as well as the profits from the operations of Freeland Hospital. In only 10 years, the foundation had accumulated $7 million. Expenditures were used largely to acquire capital equipment for Freeland Hospital.

Occasionally in the past, some members of the board of trustees had raised questions about social consciousness. The suggestion made most often was that Freeland ought to establish some outpatient clinics in areas of the adjacent city where primary care was virtually absent. Shurmann assiduously avoided taking any action on these informal recommendations.

Shurmann had recently hired a director of marketing, Maureen O'Riley, and asked her to identify some new initiatives for Freeland. O'Riley's market research resulted in a plan that included programs for respite care, addiction treatment, and rehabilitation medicine. O'Riley noted that there were no competing programs in the service area, and that the expected high level of demand would be covered by individuals or nongovernmental third party payors, both of whom were likely to pay their charges. Shurmann was enthusiastic about the suggestions and sent the proposals to the board for review.

Shurmann was shocked when his proposal ran into a brick wall at the board. No member of the board disputed the well-documented need and the potential demand for the proposed programs. They were troubled, however, by the prospect of generating additional revenues and adding them to the endowment. Several board members indicated that they would vote to approve the new programs only if a major part of any surpluses generated were used to assist the underserved areas of the city. The issue went unresolved at the meeting.

Shurmann was angry as he left the meeting, but was careful not to show his frame of mind to the board. When he had had a few minutes to reflect on the meeting, he asked his chief operating officer (COO) to come to his office. Shurmann told the COO what had happened and asked her to solicit any equipment requests that members of the medical staff might have and to have them in his office within the week. He told the COO to dust off the plans that had been developed several years earlier to build a staff education wing and the more recent request from the oncology department for an expanded unit. As the COO left, Shurmann thought to himself that he'd be damned if he'd see his hard work and fiscal success wasted on a hare-brained scheme to provide primary care to a population that should be somebody else's concern.

Freeland Hospital is wealthy, and is likely to become wealthier. The board has begun to recognize a broader social responsibility, while Shurmann sees Freeland's role as narrower. The questions raised by the board should have been addressed in the hospital's philosophy and mission statement, and these documents should be reviewed for guidance. If, however, no attention has been given to Freeland's broader social responsibility, this fundamental question must be addressed before any decisions are made on the marketing plan and the programs that have been recommended for establishment. To proceed without establishing a clear direction for the hospital would be folly.

The most powerful argument to be made opposing the board's interest in aiding the underserved areas of the city is that of service area. Given the facts, it seems likely that the city is out of Freeland's service area. It is unfair to take resources reaped from Freeland's service area and redirect them to patients outside the service area, however compelling the reason. Under this view, Freeland should reduce its surpluses (and benefit its service area) by reducing charges. This would directly benefit those whom it serves. Alternatively, Freeland could identify health needs that are not well insured, or are not likely to be highly sought by private payors, but are important health needs, nonetheless. Examples of such needs include mental health programs and various types of counseling services.

Shurmann's attitude seems excessively parochial, while the board's attitude may be excessively altruistic. There is a wide middle ground that could accommodate both. It seems more than reasonable at least to study what role Freeland could play in meeting the health needs of the wider community, whether or not it is in Freeland's service area. Additional information may make the answer very apparent.

Historical attitudes about competition, lack of profit motive, and not-for-profit status have both helped and hindered the health services system. The absence of economic incentives has contributed to health services organizations feeling good about themselves because they were doing good, rather than concentrating on performing well and efficiently. Important as a contributing factor was the fact that government programs, primarily Medicare, reimbursed providers their costs, thus rewarding the inefficient.

CONCLUSION

The competitive environment in the health services field brought with it a perceived need to market. During the 1980s, health services organizations almost universally engaged in some marketing, at least at the level of building name recognition. Especially for not-for-profit organizations, the question of whether to market raised a host of ethical issues that began with the basic question of the propriety of marketing itself, and extended to issues such as creating demand and distinguishing among various types of demand.

Hospitals with large amounts of uncompensated care may see offering better reimbursed services, such as rehabilitation and cosmetic surgery, as one way to offset these losses. "No money, no mission" is an oft-repeated justification for such actions, if one is needed. More fiscally sound hospitals must ask themselves whether they are meeting a general duty under the principle of justice to offer unprofitable but needed services that benefit the wider community.

As with all activities undertaken by the health services organization, the organizational philosophy and mission statement must provide an ethical context for marketing. Managers have a duty under the principle of respect for persons to be honest and keep the promises made in their marketing. The principle of justice suggests that careful attention must be paid to the groups and medical conditions at which marketing is focused. Non-HMO health services organizations potentially have the same ethical problems as those suggested for HMOs in Chapter 8.

NOTES

1. Robert M. Cunningham, Jr., "Of Snake Oil and Science," *Trustee 31,* no. 4 (April 1978): 34–36.

2. Victor Cohn, "Study Says Some Coronary Bypasses are Unneeded," *Washington Post,* October 27, 1983.

3. American Hospital Association, "Guidelines: Advertising by Hospitals," 1977.

4. American Hospital Association, Press Release, February 6, 1984.

5. Thomas G. Rundall, Wendy K. Lambert, and Shoshanna S. Churgin, "Hospital Deductions from Revenue in California," Western Consortium for the Health Professions, Inc., and Western Center for Health Planning, July, 1985.

6. Bradford H. Gray and Walter J. McNerney, "For-Profit Enterprise in Health Care: The Institute of Medicine Study," *New England Journal of Medicine 314,* no. 23 (June 1986): 1523–1528.

7. Barbara Arrington and Cynthia Carter Haddock, "Who *Really* Profits from Not-for-Profits?" *Health Services Research 25,* no. 2 (June 1990): 291–304.

8. American Hospital Association, *State of the Nation's Access to Hospital Services,* 4th ed. (January 1990): 2.

13

∞

DEALING WITH AIDS
A BIOMEDICAL ISSUE

THE VIRUS THAT CAUSES acquired immunodeficiency syndrome (AIDS) has proved to be an elusive foe. A great deal has been learned about the virus since it was first identified in the early 1980s, but its spread continues. Both the pessimistic prediction of a major outbreak in the general population and the optimistic prediction of it being confined to and then eliminated within the homosexual population have proved to be wrong. There have been scientific breakthroughs in understanding the virus, but there is no cure or vaccine. A second strain of the virus was isolated in the late 1980s and it is probable there will be others. Work on a vaccine has been tempered by the knowledge that rapid mutation of the AIDS virus makes developing a vaccine with long-term effectiveness difficult, if not impossible. Even if a successful vaccine were developed, it would take 5 years or more before testing and clinical trials were completed and the vaccine made available to the general population. Recently, there has been reason for cautious optimism about a vaccine, however. Three separate studies showed that monkeys vaccinated with the simian equivalent of human immunosuppressive virus (HIV) are immune from infection. In addition, seven different human vaccines have been tested.[1] Meanwhile, prevention and education have received attention unprecedented in the history of modern public health.

INCIDENCE AND PREVALENCE

A total of 102,621 cases of AIDS has been reported since June, 1981, with a fatality rate of 58%, a rate among the highest of all diseases.[2] Although drugs and improved treatment regimens have increased the life expectancy of persons with AIDS (PWAs), the outlook for long-term survival is not very bright.

According to the Centers for Disease Control (CDC), 390,000–480,000 cases of AIDS will have been reported by 1993. It is estimated that 800,000–1.2 million Americans are already infected with HIV and will eventually require care.[3] In mid-1990, the World Health Organization reported that the AIDS epidemic is accelerating dramatically and that there may be as many as 8–10 million infected people worldwide.[4] AIDS is a modern pandemic.

Nevertheless, the major outbreak of AIDS in the U.S. population that was predicted early in the epidemic has not occurred. There is, however, rapid spread of the virus among some groups. Among intravenous drug users, the incidence of AIDS is very high. The number of new cases is also rising rapidly among Hispanics and blacks. These cases are significant in and of themselves and because they place more of society at risk by spreading the virus. Conversely, the incidence of HIV among male homosexuals has slowed considerably, apparently because of changed sexual practices.

The spread of AIDS among college students is also troubling. A recent study of college students showed an average prevalence rate (existing infections) of 0.20%, with some campuses experiencing rates as high as 0.40%.[5] This means that on average 1 in 500 college students is HIV positive. At the higher level, 2 in 500 are HIV positive. The average prevalence rate for college students is higher than that among military recruits, among whom 0.14% are HIV positive. (Undoubtedly there is a significant element of self-selection in the military, because HIV-positive individuals are less likely to seek military service.) The methodology of the study of college students has been challenged and additional research is needed. The data are of great concern, however, because they suggest that college students may not be taking the risk of AIDS seriously.

RESEARCH AND TREATMENT

The federal government spent over $1.3 billion dollars on AIDS and HIV research, education, and prevention in 1989. This is more than was spent on heart disease and slightly less than was spent on cancer.[6] In addition, a great deal of research is being conducted in the private sector. Pharmaceutical companies are working hard to develop drugs to prevent HIV infection and to treat AIDS. The result will be significant improvements in the ability to treat or perhaps even to prevent the spread of the disease. New drugs are proving effective in unique ways: blocking the virus's ability to reproduce its genes, blocking the virus from multiplying in the cells, hindering a virus enzyme needed to process key viral proteins, and stimulating the immune system. There appears to be a growing sense that combinations of drugs will make AIDS a chronic rather than an acute disease.[7]

PWAs are living longer as a result of more effective medical management and healthier lifestyles, including better nutrition, and preventive measures that reduce the risk of reinfection. The drug AZT has proved effective in slowing progression of the infection, and the manufacturer recently reduced its high cost, which will increase its availability. There is preliminary evidence, however, that HIV becomes resistant to AZT. Aerosol pentamidine can be used to treat the serious pulmonary infections that afflict AIDS patients in the final phases of the disease. Neither AZT nor pentamidine cures AIDS, however.

Political and social pressures from PWAs and their supporters have caused radical changes in how the Food and Drug Administration (FDA) approves drugs to treat AIDS. Primarily, the changes mean that clinical trials are less rigorous and that the usual safety concerns receive less attention if preliminary results suggest that a drug is effective. In addition, the FDA has approved "community testing" rather than limiting clinical trials to hospitals, as it has in the past.

IMPLICATIONS OF AIDS
FOR THE HEALTH SERVICES ORGANIZATION

Financial Implications

A recent study estimated the lifetime median cost of treating a PWA to be about $24,000.[8] Other studies place the figure at $60,000 and $75,000.[9] Even the higher estimates are much lower than estimates made several years ago. It is estimated that the cumulative medical costs of treating all PWAs in the United States from the time of diagnosis until death will total $7.8 billion by 1993.[10]

The economic and social burdens of treating PWAs are inequitably distributed because of the concentration of PWAs in inner city hospitals in major metropolitan areas.[11] In its early phase, when the AIDS epidemic primarily affected the middle class, patients usually had ample insurance, although insurance coverage was often lost once the patient was unable to work. Medicaid (or Medicare, if the patient could be classified as disabled) covered medical expenses once the patient's assets had been depleted. As the demographics of the epidemic have changed, however, the number of uninsured patients has increased dramatically: PWAs are, or almost always become, uninsured. This has major implications for the economic survival of hospitals and other health services organizations, especially nursing facilities (NFs) and hospices.

Some commentators have attributed the decline in medical school applications to a concern about treating PWAs. Treating large numbers of PWAs may also affect medical residency programs. If residents cannot gain experience with a wide range of illnesses, approval for the residency may be withdrawn. Concentrations of PWAs may cause special problems for other types of staffing as well.

The geographic distribution of PWAs may be changing. PWAs will be distributed more evenly, and health services organizations nationwide will be affected. Recently, providers other than hospitals, including NFs, hospices, and home care, have been shown effective in treating PWAs and, increasingly, they are becoming sources of care. This should reduce costs and deliver care in more appropriate settings.

Financing care for PWAs is difficult for the health services organization because so much of what happens lies outside its control. Hospitals cannot refuse emergency treatment to people in need of help who show up at the emergency room. Yet, if it is to carry out its mission of providing health services, the organization must survive. The organization must set limits on the amount of uncompensated care it will provide. Based on even a limited duty of beneficence, however, the organization is obliged to provide services that assist all groups and to serve as a resource to the community. The governing body and the organization's managers should develop a mission statement and policies that reflect this commitment. Some organizations chose to offer services that generate surpluses that are used to subsidize uncompensated care and fund programs for the underserved. Although laudable in their intent and end result, these efforts raise other ethical questions, such as creating demand for marginally needed services.

The dispersion of PWAs to nonurban, low-incidence areas of the country will spread the social and economic burdens of AIDS and will bring a measure of relief to urban hospitals. These hospitals are likely to continue to suffer greatly from the financial consequences of AIDS, however. No solutions are apparent, except to fund treatment through public programs such as Medicare and Medicaid. This will be fair only if funding levels are sufficient to give the organizations the reimbursement levels needed to survive. Society cannot escape the heavy economic burdens lying ahead, however, regardless of how the care is funded. In Houston, the bankruptcy in 1987 of the only dedicated AIDS hospital added to the anxiety felt by all health services managers, even though low occupancy because of few referrals was the apparent cause of that failure.

Legal Implications

The legal dimensions of AIDS are complex. The number of AIDS-related lawsuits is larger than that attributable to any other single disease in U.S. legal history, and it is predicted that health services organizations will become the most important area of AIDS-related litigation in the next few years.[12]

The Occupational Safety and Health Act administered by the Occupational Safety and Health Administration (OSHA) requires that employers provide employment and a place of employment that are free from recognized hazards that cause, or are likely to cause, death or serious physical harm. Universal blood and body substance precautions are required by OSHA. Such precautions are likely to be the focus of enforcement that will use a targeted basis (e.g., industry, type of provider) as well as responding to employee complaints. OSHA is also expected to require employee educational programs about hazards and precautions, and to engage in its own educational activities.

The second legal dimension concerns the risk to patients and staff from HIV-infected employees. Health services organizations are subject to Section 504 of the federal Rehabilitation Act of 1973, which requires that employers may not discriminate on the basis of handicap. Complementary state legislation may exist as well. The Supreme Court recently considered a situation analogous to that of an HIV-positive employee. In *Arline v. School Board of Nassau County, Florida,* a teacher who had had three recurrences of tuberculosis was discharged because the school board considered her a health threat to students. The Court ruled that the teacher's disease was a handicap protected by the statute. The case was remanded for the trial court to determine whether Arline was otherwise qualified, and whether she could have been accommodated in alternative employment.

In *Arline,* the Court stated (in a footnote) that it was not making a determination as to whether carriers of a contagious disease such as AIDS would be considered to have a physical impairment, or whether they would be considered handicapped under the act solely on the basis of contagiousness. Several important factors will affect the legal rights of an employee with AIDS. These include: the state of the disease (chronic versus acute), the type of setting in which the employee works, the risk to healthy people (as in the *Arline* case) versus the risk to ill non-AIDS patients, and the established legal duties health services organizations owe patients. HIV-positive employees may also be treated differently from employees with AIDS. Early cases have held that AIDS is a handicap within the meaning of Section 504 of the federal Rehabilitation Act of 1973 and similar state statutes. Additional protection for those who are HIV positive is found in the Civil Rights Restoration Action of 1988.[13]

Ethical and Administrative Implications

Recent clinical developments allow all health services organizations to treat AIDS patients more effectively. Generally, staff are better prepared and have developed specialized clinical skills. These, in addition to new drugs, will increase longevity for PWAs. The result will be more episodes of hospitalization, as well as treatment at other types of organizations, especially NFs.

The AIDS epidemic raises significant ethical issues for the organization and its managers. These issues include: 1) protecting staff providing care to infected patients, 2) protecting patients and staff from infected staff, and 3) maintaining the confidentiality of staff and patients with AIDS. All of these issues are being addressed; some are more easily solved than others.

Protecting Staff from Patients

The major premise for all of the organization's relationships is that in the presence of a significant infectious disease, the organization must do all it can to protect staff as they care for patients. This is supported by fidelity, part of the principle of respect for persons. Through its managers, the organization has a duty to provide a work place that is as safe as it can be. This duty can be based on the theory of utility—the greatest good for the greatest number—and is achievable only with an effective health services work force, which in turn is possible only if there are safe working conditions. Legal obligations also support this duty toward staff.

Having identified the ethical priority of protecting staff, it is necessary to answer the question of how to create and maintain an environment that is compatible with the obligation to provide health services to the community, as well as to treat PWAs.

Some physicians and staff are reluctant or unwilling to treat PWAs. There have been reports of surgeons who demand preoperative HIV testing of patients and refuse to operate on patients who test positive. In 1987, the American Medical Association (AMA) Council on Ethical and Judicial Affairs issued a statement that physicians behave unethically if they refuse to treat PWAs whose medical conditions are within their competence.[14] Nurses and staff have also been disciplined for refusing to treat PWAs; some have been fired. Given the nature of the issue, it is unlikely that statements such as the AMA statement or even disciplinary action by the organization will end the problem of caregivers refusing to treat PWAs.

Although the AIDS virus is present in all body substances of people who test HIV positive, AIDS can apparently be spread only by sexual intercourse or intimate contact with body substances, particularly blood. The risk for health care workers is very low, but a major concern. The CDC and OSHA have developed guidelines for universal precautions. These should be in use in all health services organizations.

In mid-1987, the American Hospital Association (AHA) issued recommendations reflecting the growing concern about clinical management of AIDS patients.[15] These recommendations were consistent with CDC guidelines that universal use of blood and body substance precautions is the best protection for caregivers. The guidelines suggest that all patients' blood and body substances be considered hazardous, and that all patients be subject to the infection-control guidelines originally established for hepatitis and active AIDS patients. This means that isolation and biohazard precautions should be used for all patients (whether or not they have AIDS), and that health care workers should protect themselves against body substances and patient contact. This approach was recommended over routine HIV testing of all patients.

A few hospitals test all admissions for HIV. Patients who refuse to be tested are admitted, but are treated with extra precautions. Using extra precautions is at variance with the requirements for universal precautions. In late 1987, the AHA spoke out against routine testing of patients or staff. It continues to hold that position.

In late August, 1987—and following CDC-confirmed AIDS infections acquired by three hospital staff who had been exposed to AIDS infected blood—the CDC revised its recommendations to allow hospitals more latitude in conducting routine AIDS testing. Since then, the CDC has confirmed 27 cases worldwide of health care workers who have become infected with HIV through occupational exposures.[16] Experts speculate that HIV among health care workers is significantly underreported.[17] Three large studies have estimated the risk of contracting the virus after accidentally being stuck with a contaminated needle at about 1 in 250.[18]

The risk of caregivers being infected by exposure to blood and body substances from HIV-positive patients is low. Nonetheless, it is troublesome that one study found high levels of noncompliance with universal precautions. A study conducted at the Johns Hopkins Hospital emergency department found that physicians complied with universal precautions requirements only 38% of the time. Residents and nurses complied more often (58% and 44% of the time, respectively). Housekeeping staff complied most often (91% of the time). Emergency department personnel blamed their lack of compliance on time pressures and interference of precautions with procedural skills.[19] These low levels of compliance occurred despite ready availability of gloves, gowns, and other protective gear, and despite efforts to educate staff about the known risks of contracting AIDS. The study also revealed that the rate of infected patients in the Johns Hopkins Hospital emergency department increased from 5.2% to 6.0% in 1 year. Encouraging compliance poses a special challenge to health services managers, and further research on how to encourage compliance needs to be done. Enhanced education can be only a small part of the answer. Caregivers must be aware of the risk of HIV and understand how that risk can be minimized. Management must identify and correct structure and process inhibitors that reduce the staff's willingness or ability to comply with requirements of universal precautions.

Health services organizations that follow CDC and AHA guidelines—the ethically and clinically correct and legally prudent course—treat all patients as if they were HIV positive. The August, 1987, CDC guidelines also suggested that hospitals must judge whether their patients' characteristics are such that all admissions should be tested. All health services organizations, but especially hospitals, NFs, and hospices, should address this question.

Protecting Patients from Staff

HIV-positive caregivers pose a risk of infection to patients and other staff. This risk comes from both HIV itself and from the opportunistic diseases that afflict PWAs, including tuberculosis and pneumocystis carinii pneumonia. Immunosuppressed patients are especially at risk. Significant, too, and much more subtle is the fact that the AIDS virus adversely affects the brain long before other symptoms appear. This greatly complicates the question of using HIV-positive staff.

The ethical (and legal) problems for health services organizations are complicated by the fact that some caregivers are HIV positive, but do not yet have active AIDS, and wish to continue treating patients. The most publicized cases have involved physicians. A Cook County Hospital physician was allowed to continue practicing, but was banned from performing invasive procedures. He brought suit, challenging the hospital's definition of invasive as too broad. The hospital board voted to reverse its decision. The physician subsequently died. In the interim, the Cook County Board, which is also the hospital board, approved a policy that allows patients to refuse to be treated by persons with HIV. It was unclear how the board would put this policy into effect.[20]

Another case occurred at Johns Hopkins Hospital, where a resident was infected when he was cut by a broken vial containing HIV-infected blood. He sued the hospital because of alleged breaches of confidentiality and defamation. A case recently settled in New York involved a physician who allegedly contracted AIDS during her internship when she jabbed herself with the needle of a syringe negligently left on a bed after it was used on an AIDS patient.

Despite the uncertainty of statutory and case law, all health services organizations should identify HIV-positive staff (including physicians). It is ethically appropriate and legally prudent to prohibit HIV-positive staff from performing invasive procedures. In meeting their ethical duty of nonmaleficence, staff themselves should want to know whether they pose a risk to patients and other staff. Because of the opportunistic diseases they contract, staff with AIDS may pose risks to patients, many of whom are immunosuppressed or physically weakened. Staff with AIDS may also pose risks to other employees and to visitors. These risks should cause managers to err in favor of caution in assigning staff, at least until legal parameters are established. Furthermore, as HIV-positive staff become increasingly immunosuppressed, infectious diseases commonly found in health services organizations will pose risks to them. If the health services organization is to discharge its ethical obligation toward its staff, it must be able to consider such information in job assignment. Given how much remains unknown about the virus and its transmissibility, HIV-positive staff should be encouraged to accept nonpatient care job assignments, whether or not they perform invasive procedures. Physicians who wish to continue to perform invasive procedures pose a special problem. Given the risk to patients, HIV-positive physicians must be prohibited from performing invasive procedures, as reasonably defined. Protecting staff confidentiality to the greatest extent possible is crucial to the success of any such effort.

An equally compelling and more subtle reason for routine testing of staff is suggested by data indicating that HIV induces neuropsychiatric problems. Manifestations include impaired coordination and cognitive difficulties, which may occur before physical symptoms are apparent. In normal clinical practice, deficits in performance may be attributed to random error rather than the result of a medical condition. It is possible that serious problems may occur before a pattern is detected; diminished competence may be apparent only in retrospect, possibly after harm has been inflicted on a patient. The ethical (and legal) duty of employers to monitor staff and prevent harm to patients is well established.

Something Must Be Done, But What?

Stunned, Carolyn Aubrey, the CEO of Metropolitan Hospital, sank into her chair and stared out the window for a very long time. She realized when Dr. Midmore's wife had angrily insisted on seeing the CEO that something was afoot. But even in her worst nightmares, Aubrey could never have imagined that Mrs. Midmore would tell Aubrey that she was suing her husband, an orthopedic surgeon, for divorce because he had given her AIDS. As Mrs. Midmore left Aubrey's office, she had turned back and said, "I was sure you'd want to know—surely you'll want to do something."

Fleetingly, Aubrey thought Mrs. Midmore's remarks might be nothing more than the ravings of an angry, vindictive wife, but that wasn't likely. As she considered what she had just learned, she recalled an incident several years ago involving Dr. Midmore and a male orderly. In retrospect, it now suggested that Dr. Midmore might be bisexual. Aubrey thought, too, about the department of surgery meeting last year when there had been a long discussion about the desirability of knowing the HIV status of all surgical patients. The special risks of torn gloves and cuts during orthopedic surgery had been described in detail.

Now it seemed that Dr. Midmore's patients were at special risk. Aubrey called operating room scheduling and learned that Dr. Midmore was maintaining a full surgical load. Aubrey asked her secretary to call the hospital attorney and the medical director and set up an emergency meeting for 7:00 the following morning. Mrs. Midmore had been right, thought Aubrey. We'll have to do something, but what?

This case touches on several ethical (and legal) issues. First, and with all possible haste, Aubrey and her staff must determine the accuracy of the information. This investigation will include questioning Dr. Midmore and confirming his wife's statements. If there is reasonable cause—thus meeting the requirements of the principle of justice (fairness)—Dr. Midmore's surgical privileges must be suspended, thus meeting the principle of nonmaleficience by preventing potential harm to patients. Once Dr. Midmore is no longer a risk to patients, further action can follow in a more orderly and deliberate manner, always, however, consistent with the need to protect patients and the requirements in the medical staff bylaws.

Confidentiality regarding Dr. Midmore's HIV status is important and everything possible must be done to safeguard it. Efforts made in this regard must never be allowed to compromise patient safety, however. The issue of confidentiality takes on further complexity if Dr. Midmore leaves the staff and applies for surgical privileges elsewhere. Should this occur, the hospital has an ethical obligation to communicate what it has learned in the course of its investigation.

Maintaining Patient Confidentiality

Health services organizations must be alert to the special problems of confidentiality when treating AIDS patients. Within the constraints of state law, however, the first obligation must be to safeguard the health of staff and other patients. Identifying HIV-positive patients may be an important additional stimulus that will encourage staff to comply with universal precautions.

It has been argued that identifying patients as HIV positive will lead to a two-class medical system. This charge is baseless. The potential for this problem has existed since HIV was first identified and patient charts and rooms were marked with biohazard notices, as well as other, less transparent codes. Thus far, there is no evidence that PWAs have received care different from that accorded other patients.

Establishing a Dedicated AIDS Unit

Dedicated units for PWAs are rare. The vast majority of health services organizations, including hospitals, have too few PWAs to justify establishing a dedicated unit. Typically, hospitals with large numbers of PWAs admit them to general medical/surgical floors rather than to dedicated units, even for acute phases of the disease. Managers argue that privacy is better protected; the extra workload is spread among caregivers, especially nurses; and staffing and work assignment problems are eased.

More dedicated AIDS units may be established as the public becomes more willing to accept PWAs and as the financial effects of AIDS become more acute. It is possible that public agencies will then establish or staff AIDS hospitals, NFs, and other types of special treatment programs.

Loss of patient confidentiality is often cited when dedicated AIDS units are discussed. This risk is overstated because staff know (as they should) which patients have AIDS. With the wide publicity AIDS has received, it is likely that family members and visitors will be aware of the possibility of AIDS, especially in the final stages of the disease. Concentrating PWAs in one unit allows special training and equipment to be brought to bear to protect staff and to enhance treatment. Moreover, it allows those staff members who wish to work with PWAs to do so. A dedicated unit also minimizes any drift toward second-class care, because the availability of staff and other resources would be readily apparent, whereas such lapses could be more easily overlooked or hidden on a general medical/surgical floor.

CONCLUSION

AIDS has ethical, legal, financial, and management dimensions and nuances that make it as complex an issue as managers are likely to see. Caring for PWAs while protecting staff remains a major ethical and legal challenge, and one in which managers will play the leading role.

AIDS continues to represent a major threat to society, even though changes in sexual practices and use of preventive measures have proved effective in dramatically slowing the spread of HIV among one high-risk group, male homosexuals. The challenge is to find ways to encourage other high-risk groups—including intravenous drug users, minority populations, and a new group, college students—to protect themselves against infection.

Hospitals must find ways to provide effective acute, episodic treatment and to assist health services organizations, especially NFs and hospices, that provide alternative sources of care. Financing care will remain problematic for all providers.

Encouraging in the effort to solve the health problems associated with AIDS is the fact that the debate has become less hysterical. There is an increasing willingness to treat AIDS as primarily a public health problem with political and civil rights dimensions, rather than as primarily a political and civil rights problem with public health dimensions.

Most disconcerting for both the near- and long-term is that the public has turned its attention elsewhere. The major reason for this loss of interest is that the epidemic has been milder than predicted several years ago. Psychologically, it is yesterday's news. Health services organizations are seeking a just solution to financing care for the underserved and uninsured; lack of public attention, however, will make this task more difficult, if not impossible.

NOTES

1. Larry Thompson, "Vaccines: A Status Report," *Washington Post*, Health Section, April 3, 1990.

2. Gail Friedman, "Hospital Growing AIDS Care is Bumping Other Services," *HealthWeek*, August 28, 1989, 5.

3. "Estimates of HIV Prevalence and Projected AIDS Cases: Summary of a Workshop, October 31–November 1, 1989," *Morbidity and Mortality Weekly Review 39*, no. 7 (February 23, 1990): 110–112, 117–119.

4. Malcolm Gladwell, "AIDS Spreading 'Dramatically' Worldwide," *Washington Post*, August 1, 1990.

5. Susan Okie, "HIV Infection Found in 1 of 500 College Students," *Washington Post*, May 23, 1989.

6. William Winkenwerder, Austin R. Kessler, and Rhonda M. Stolec, "Federal Spending for Illness Caused by the Human Immunodeficiency Virus," *New England Journal of Medicine 320*, no. 24 (June 1989): 1602.

7. Larry Thompson, "New Treatments: Drug Combinations Might Hobble AIDS Virus," *Washington Post*, Health Section, April 3, 1990.

8. Joel W. Hay, "Projecting the Medical Costs of HIV/AIDS: An Update with Focus on Epidemiology," *New Perspectives on HIV-Related Illnesses: Progress in Health Services Research*. Proceedings of a conference sponsored by the National Center for Health Services Research and Health Care Technology Assessment, Public Health Service, Department of Health and Human Services, DHHS Publication No. (PHS) 89-3449 (September 1989): 84–85.

9. Hay, "Projecting Medical Costs of HIV/AIDS"; Department of Health and Human Services, Public Health Service, "Cumulative Costs of Treating AIDS Are Estimated," *Research Activities*, Agency for Health Care Policy and Research, no. 126 (February 1990): 5.

10. Department of Health and Human Services, Public Health Service, "Cumulative Costs of Treating AIDS."

11. Sandra G. Boodman, "Up Against It: In Newark, A Public Hospital Fights the Twin Plagues of AIDS and Drugs," *Washington Post*, Health Section, September 5, 1989; "AIDS Update: An Executive Report," *Hospitals* (May 5, 1990): 26–34.

12. "AIDS-Related Lawsuits Will Continue to Rise, Report Shows," *AHA News*, April 16, 1990.

13. "HIV-Infected Physicians and the Practice of Seriously Invasive Procedures," *Hastings Center Report 19*, no. 1 (January/February 1989): 37.

14. American Medical Association, "Ethical Issues Involved in the Growing AIDS Crisis," *Reports of the Council on Ethical and Judicial Affairs* (December 1987). The report states that "A physician who knows that he or she has an infectious disease should not engage in any activity that creates a risk of transmission of the disease to others. . . . disclosure of that risk to patients is not enough; patients are entitled to expect that their physicians will not increase their exposure to the risk of contracting an infectious disease, even minimally".

15. American Hospital Association, *AIDS/HIV Infection: Recommendations for Health Care Practices and Public Policy, Report and Recommendations of the Special Committee on AIDS/HIV Infection Policy, 1987–1988*.

16. Jeffrey Green, "Prego AIDS Case: Settlement Leaves Few Answers for Hospitals," *AHA News,* March 19, 1990.

17. Susan Okie, "HIV-Infected Workers Undercounted," *Washington Post,* January 16, 1990.

18. Ibid.

19. Mary Koska, "AIDS Precautions: Compliance Difficult to Enforce," *Hospitals* (September 5, 1989): 58.

20. "Chicago Patients Gain Curb on AIDS Carriers," *New York Times,* September 22, 1988.

ORGANIZATIONAL PHILOSOPHIES AND MISSION STATEMENTS

Philosophy of the Franciscan Health System

We, the Sisters of St. Francis of Philadelphia, welcome all of God's people as sisters and brothers in the spirit of St. Francis of Assisi. Our desire to live the gospel impels us to serve in the ministry of health care with compassion and courage, trusting in the loving providence of God.

We believe that because all persons are created in God's own likeness, we are all members of one human family through God's Son and our Brother, Jesus. In every dimension of our health care ministry we witness to the inherent dignity of human life. While utilizing the technological resources of modern science, we give priority to the creation of a community environment which fosters human dignity and relationships.

Therefore, through the Franciscan Health System we commit ourselves to these beliefs:

HUMAN LIFE

> Reverencing all human life as a precious gift of the Creator, we refrain from all that threatens or diminishes life both before and after birth, and, despite sickness, disabilities and handicaps, we cherish and protect life until the moment of death.

WHOLISM

> We recognize that the development and integration of all facets of the human person are necessary for health and wellness. We promote the concept of wholism in all our health care endeavors, both for those served by us and those associated with us in ministry.

SHARED MINISTRY

> We highly value the laity who co-minister with us, acknowledging with gratitude their contribution to the healing ministry of Jesus. We seek to affirm and encourage them as they continue to assume greater responsibility and leadership in this ministry.

PEACEMAKING

As Franciscan peacemakers, we actively work for a just and peaceful world. We reject all forms of injustice and anything that results in harm or violence to the human person, to human relationships or to the environment.

Mission Statement of Saint Mary Hospital

Empowered by the Spirit of JESUS CHRIST and inspired by the examples of Saint Francis of Assisi, Saint John Neumann, Mother Francis Bachmann and the Sisters of Saint Francis of Philadelphia, we manifest our participation in the healing ministry of the Roman Catholic Church through our commitment to provide, within the limits of our resources, compassionate and quality holistic care to all in our community, within which we especially cherish the poor. We envision that the scope of the healing ministry will become more expansive and varied. Therefore, we will endeavor to accept, discover and create new structures, models and services to enhance health care at Saint Mary Hospital of Langhorne.

From Saint Mary Hospital, Langhorne, PA, 1990; reprinted with permission.

Mission Statement of Riverside Medical Center

The missions of Fairview and Carondelet LifeCare Corporation shall be implemented through Riverside Medical Center. Riverside Medical Center shall carry on the healing ministry of Jesus Christ to provide quality health care services. This service of health care respects individual beliefs in a spirit of Christian concern and is given to the people in the communities that we serve. The relationship embodies the ecumenical bond of the Catholic and Lutheran constituencies.

In fulfillment of this mission, we affirm that Riverside Medical Center:

1. Shall be a consolidated campus with an integrated board, management structure and medical staff which allows two existing organizations to maintain their own particular philosophy of health care. Each member of Riverside Medical Center will have the ability to maintain its own medical/ethical positions in light of its own religious traditions and yet have a consistent approach to the ethical problems they share in common.
2. Shall encompass concern for the whole person and be committed to care for body, mind and spirit.
3. Shall regard people we serve as persons of dignity and worth.
4. Shall make professional excellence paramount by meeting or surpassing established community standards for quality care.
5. Shall emphasize care to the poor and underserved in cooperation with other community providers and within Riverside Medical Center's ability to provide support.
6. Shall nurture high ethical standards and recognize the value of each employee in fulfilling the mission of Riverside Medical Center.
7. Shall maintain open communication and relationships of trust, respect and concern among employees, physicians, board members and volunteers to provide an environment for personal satisfaction, growth and effectiveness.
8. Shall promote equity and fundamental fairness in all organizational transactions.
9. Shall foster personal innovation and organizational creativity.
10. Shall participate in and carry on research and education activities supportive to its mission.

From Riverside Medical Center, Minneapolis, MN; reprinted with permission.

Mission Statement of Adventist Health System

Our Mission   The Seventh-day Adventist philosophy of healthcare is based on the belief that God originally created man in His image. Man, through separation from God, has suffered physical, mental, and spiritual damage. Shady Grove's goal is to bring healing to man through a ministry of kindness, understanding, and love.

Our Patients   This ministry affects every aspect of Shady Grove's operation, especially patient care. At Shady Grove, patients are treated as guests of the hospital family. Our employees strive to understand patients' physical, emotional, and spiritual needs, and impart Judeo-Christian love.

Shady Grove's commitment to excellence in modern medicine is an intrinsic part of our goal of healing for the body, mind, and spirit. This commitment places us at the forefront of modern healthcare. We combine a staff of carefully selected healthcare professionals with the latest technological advances to provide the finest medical care for our community.

In addition to treatment, healing involves education and prevention. Members of the hospital staff emphasize principles of healthful living, guiding patients, their families, and friends toward a healthier lifestyle.

Shady Grove recognizes that the rapidly changing healthcare environment creates increasingly complex bio-ethical issues. Each doctor, patient, and patient's family work as a team to thoughtfully consider medical decisions. We have established a committee of physicians and other healthcare professionals to carefully consider ethical issues as they affect hospital policies and a patient's freedom of choice.

While it is our philosophy of healing that gives our ministry meaning, it is the financial stability of our hospital that makes this ministry possible. As a not-for-profit hospital, we strive to increase the quality of our service through wise and ethical management of financial, material, and human resources.

Our Employees   Because the ministry of kindness begins with our own employees, Shady Grove values the physical, emotional, and spiritual well-being of each employee.

As an important member of the hospital family, each employee shares the responsibility for creating an atmosphere of love and kindness at Shady Grove. All departments are encouraged to work together as a team for better patient care, a better working environment, and a stronger hospital.

Our Community Shady Grove is a place where all members of our community can feel welcome. As a community hospital, we respect the spiritual, cultural, and social diversities our patients, physicians, and community cherish.

We treasure our active involvement with the community we serve and vigorously seek to extend that involvement. We value the support of the many volunteers and contributors who have helped build and maintain Shady Grove.

Each department at Shady Grove strives to serve the community, an integral part of the ministry of kindness at Shady Grove Adventist Hospital.

Mission and Purpose Statement of
The George Washington University Health Plan

GWUHP was organized on May 16, 1972, as a not-for-profit corporation in the District of Columbia. The purpose of the Corporation, as stated in its Articles of Incorporation, include the following:

(a)   To advance the development of comprehensive health care and to promote medical education by formulating a program or programs of prepaid comprehensive health services for a subscribing population;

(b)   To contract with hospitals, group medical clinics, nursing homes and other corporations, persons and individuals qualified or licensed to render health care services or licensed to practice medicine in any and all forms;

(c)   To provide patient care, to engage in teaching and research and to perform services and engage in activities incidental thereto; and

(d)   To establish, operate and maintain medical service centers and such other facilities as may aid in the study, prevention, diagnosis, care and treatment of human ailments and injuries.

From The George Washington University Health Plan, Washington, DC, 1972; reprinted with permission.

Mission Statement of the
Hebrew Home of Greater Washington

1. Working Assumptions

   a. The Washington Jewish community, one of the largest Jewish communities in the United States, has the will and the means to support a model geriatric institution, which can be a national leader in the care of the elderly. Jewish geriatric facilities in many other large cities have taken the lead in offering a combination of institutional, residential and community services for the elderly. The Hebrew Home of Greater Washington is committed to being a national leader in providing innovative and exemplary care to the elderly. This commitment extends to teaching, research and the furtherance of knowledge in long-term care.

   b. Elderly Jews in the Greater Washington community should have access to quality health care, regardless of their ability to pay for that care.

   c. In the future, the health care needs for the dependent elderly housed at the Hebrew Home will be more acute, complex and intense. As the Jewish elderly population increases, the housing and care needs of the independent frail elderly will become greater. There will be need for an array of coordinated health and social services provided at home or in clustered sheltered housing to people who might have become residents of the Home in the past.

   d. The current facilities and programs of the Home will be inadequate to meet the projected needs. Care in the future need not be exclusively limited to residential care at the Rockville campus. New ways of economically and efficiently delivering services to meet the community's needs should be identified, planned and provided.

2. Mission Statement

   The mission of the Hebrew Home of Greater Washington is to fulfill the Jewish value of providing care for the elderly while respecting Jewish cultural ideas and traditions.

   The Hebrew Home of Greater Washington is committed to providing and coordinating exemplary health care, housing and supportive services for Jewish elderly. The Home's first priority is to serve the most dependent elderly; however, it recognizes a responsibility to care for those whose level of independence is decreasing and to plan and provide for their long-term needs.

To the extent that gaps exist between needs of the elderly and services provided by public and private agencies, the Home will provide services, encourage the provision of new services by other organizations or assist in the coordination of newer services provided by other agencies.

The Hebrew Home respects and appreciates the important contributions made by other agencies of the Jewish community, values the assistance the community receives from these agencies, and will, in the course of fulfilling this mission statement, seek to coordinate its programs with Jewish community agencies serving the elderly.

ETHICAL CODES

American College of Healthcare Executives (ACHE) Code of Ethics

PREAMBLE

The purpose of the Code of Ethics of the American College of Healthcare Executives is to serve as a guide to conduct for affiliates. It contains standards of ethical behavior for healthcare executives in their professional relationships. These relationships include members of the healthcare executive's organization and other organizations. Also included are patients, clients or others served, colleagues, the community and society as a whole. The Code of Ethics also incorporates standards of ethical behavior governing personal behavior, particularly when that conduct directly relates to the role and identity of the healthcare executive.

The fundamental objectives of the healthcare management profession are to enhance overall quality of life, dignity and well-being of every individual needing healthcare services; and to create a more equitable, accessible, effective and efficient healthcare system.

Healthcare executives have an obligation to act in ways that will merit the trust, confidence and respect of healthcare professionals and the general public. To do so, healthcare executives must lead lives that embody an exemplary system of values and ethics.

In fulfilling their commitments and obligations to patients, clients or others they serve, healthcare executives function as moral agents. Since every management decision affects the health and well-being of both individuals and communities, healthcare executives must evaluate the possible outcomes of their decisions and accept full responsibility for the consequences. In organizations that deliver healthcare services, they must safeguard and foster the rights, interests and prerogatives of patients, clients or others served. The role of moral agent requires that healthcare executives speak out and take actions necessary to promote such rights, interests and prerogatives if they are threatened.

I. THE HEALTHCARE EXECUTIVE'S RESPONSIBILITIES TO THE PROFESSION OF HEALTHCARE MANAGEMENT
    The healthcare executive shall:

A. Uphold the values, ethics and mission of the healthcare management profession;

B. Conduct all personal and professional activities with honesty, integrity, respect, fairness and good faith in a manner that will reflect well upon the profession;

C. Comply with all laws in the jurisdictions in which the healthcare executive is located, or conducts professional or personal activities;

D. Maintain competence and proficiency in healthcare management by implementing a personal program of assessment and continuing professional education;

E. Avoid the exploitation of professional relationships for personal gain;

F. Use this code to further the interests of the profession and not for selfish reasons;

G. Respect professional confidences;

H. Enhance the dignity and image of the healthcare management profession through positive public information programs;

I. Refrain from participating in any endorsement or publicity that demeans the credibility and dignity of the healthcare management profession; and

J. Refrain from using the College's credential or affiliation with the College to promote or endorse external commercial products or services.

II. THE HEALTHCARE EXECUTIVE'S OBLIGATIONS TO THE ORGANIZATION AND TO PATIENTS, CLIENTS OR OTHERS SERVED

A. COMMITMENTS TO THE ORGANIZATION

1. Provide healthcare services consistent with available resources and assure the existence of a resource allocation process that considers ethical ramifications;

2. Conduct both comprehensive and cooperative activities in ways that improve community healthcare services;

3. Lead the organization in the use and improvement of standards of management and sound business practices;

4. Respect the customs and practices of patients, clients or others served, consistent with the organization's philosophy; and

5. Be truthful in all forms of professional and organizational communication and avoid information that is false, misleading, and deceptive or information that would create unreasonable expectations.

B. COMMITMENTS TO PATIENTS, CLIENTS OR OTHERS SERVED
The healthcare executive shall:

1. Assure the existence of a process to evaluate the quality of care or service rendered;

2. Avoid exploitation of relationships for personal advantage;

3. Avoid practicing or facilitating discrimination and institute safeguards to prevent discriminatory organizational practices;

4. Assure the existence of a process that will advise patients, clients or others served of the rights, opportunities, responsibilities and risks regarding available healthcare services;

5. Provide a process which assures the autonomy and self-determination of patients, clients or others served, and

6. Assure the existence of procedures that will safeguard the confidentiality and privacy of patients, clients and others served.

C. CONFLICTS OF INTEREST
A conflict of interest may be only a matter of degree, but exists when the healthcare executive

- is in a position to benefit directly or indirectly by using authority or inside information, or allows a friend, relative or associate to benefit from such authority or information.

- uses authority or information to make a decision to intentionally affect the organization in an adverse manner.

The healthcare executive shall:

1. Conduct all personal and professional relationships in such a way that all those affected are assured that management decisions are made in the best interests of the organization and the individuals served by it;

2. Disclose to the appropriate authority any direct or indirect financial or personal interests that might pose potential conflicts of interest;

3. Accept no gifts or benefits offered with the expectation of influencing a management decision; and

4. Inform the appropriate authority and other involved parties of potential conflicts of interest related to appointments or elections to boards or committees inside or outside the healthcare executive's organization.

III. THE HEALTHCARE EXECUTIVE'S RESPONSIBILITIES TO COMMUNITY AND SOCIETY
The healthcare executive shall:

A. Work to identify and meet the healthcare needs of the community;

B. Work to assure that all people have reasonable access to healthcare services;

C. Participate in public dialogue on healthcare policy issues and advocate solutions that will improve health status and promote quality healthcare;

D. Consider the short-term and long-term impact of management decisions on both the community and on society; and

E. Provide prospective consumers with adequate and accurate information, enabling them to make enlightened judgments and decisions regarding services.

IV. THE HEALTHCARE EXECUTIVE'S DUTY TO REPORT VIOLATIONS OF THE CODE

An affiliate of the College who has reasonable grounds to believe that another affiliate has violated this Code has a duty to communicate such facts to the Committee on Ethics.

From American College of Healthcare Executives, "Codes of Ethics," 1988, reprinted with permission.

American College of Health Care Administrators (ACHCA) Code of Ethics

PREAMBLE

The preservation of the highest standards of integrity and ethical principles is vital to the successful discharge of the professional responsibilities of all long-term health care administrators. This Code of Ethics has been promulgated by the American College of Health Care Administrators (ACHCA) in an effort to stress the fundamental rules considered essential to this basic purpose. It shall be the obligation of members to seek to avoid not only conduct specifically proscribed by the code, but also conduct that is inconsistent with its spirit and purpose. Failure to specify any particular responsibility or practice in this Code of Ethics should not be construed as denial of the existence of other responsibilities or practices. Recognizing that the ultimate responsibility for applying standards and ethics falls upon the individual, the ACHCA establishes the following Code of Ethics to make clear its expectation of the membership.

EXPECTATION I—Individuals shall hold paramount the welfare of persons for whom care is provided.

PRESCRIPTIONS: The Health Care Administrator shall:

Strive to provide to all those entrusted to his or her care the highest quality of appropriate services possible in light of resources or other constraints.

Operate the facility consistent with laws, regulations and standards of practice recognized in the field of health care administration.

Consistent with law and professional standards, protect the confidentiality of information regarding individual recipients of care.

Perform administrative duties with the personal integrity that will earn the confidence, trust, and respect of the general public.

Take appropriate steps to avoid discrimination on basis of race, color, sex, religion, age, national origin, handicap, marital status, ancestry, or any other factor that is illegally discriminatory or not related to bona fide requirements of quality care.

PROSCRIPTIONS: The Health Care Administrator shall *not*:

Disclose professional or personal information regarding recipients of service to unauthorized personnel unless required by law or to protect the public welfare.

EXPECTATION II—Individuals shall maintain high standards of professional competence.

PRESCRIPTIONS: The Health Care Administrator shall:

Possess and maintain the competencies necessary to effectively perform his or her responsibilities.

Practice administration in accordance with capabilities and proficiencies and, when appropriate, seek counsel from qualified others.

Actively strive to enhance knowledge of and expertise in long-term care administration through continuing education and professional development.

PROSCRIPTIONS: The Health Care Administrator shall *not*:

Misrepresent qualifications, education, experience, or affiliations.

Provide services other than those for which he or she is prepared and qualified to perform.

EXPECTATION III—Individuals shall strive in all matters relating to their professional functions, to maintain a professional posture that places paramount the interests of the facility and its residents.

PRESCRIPTIONS: The Health Care Administrator shall:

Avoid partisanship and provide a forum for the fair resolution of any disputes which may arise in service delivery or facility management.

Disclose to the governing body or other authority as may be appropriate, any actual or potential circumstance concerning him or her that might reasonably be thought to create a conflict of interest or have a substantial adverse impact on the facility or its residents.

PROSCRIPTION: The Health Care Administrator shall *not*:

Participate in activities that reasonably may be thought to create a conflict of interest or have the potential to have a substantial adverse impact on the facility or its residents.

EXPECTATION IV—Individuals shall honor their responsibilities to the public, their profession, and their relationships with colleagues and members of related professions.

PRESCRIPTIONS: The Health Care Administrator shall:

Foster increased knowledge within the profession of health care administration and support research efforts toward this end.

Participate with others in the community to plan for and provide a full range of health care services.

Share areas of expertise with colleagues, students and the general public to increase awareness and promote understanding of health care in general and the profession in particular.

Inform the ACHCA Standards and Ethics Committee of actual or potential violations of this Code of Ethics, and fully cooperate with ACHCA's sanctioned inquiries into matters of professional conduct related to this Code of Ethics.

PROSCRIPTION: The Health Care Administrator shall *not*:

Defend, support or ignore unethical conduct perpetrated by colleagues, peers, or students.

From American College of Health Care Administrators, "Code of Ethics," 1989, reprinted with permission.

American Medical Association (AMA) Principles of Medical Ethics

PREAMBLE

The medical profession has long subscribed to a body of ethical statements developed primarily for the benefit of the patient. As a member of this profession, a physician must recognize responsibility not only to patients, but also to society, to other health professionals, and to self. The following Principles adopted by the American Medical Association are not laws, but standards of conduct which define the essentials of honorable behavior for the physician.

I. A physician shall be dedicated to providing competent medical service with compassion and respect for human dignity.

II. A physician shall deal honestly with patient and colleagues, and strive to expose those physicians deficient in character or competence, or who engage in fraud or deception.

III. A physician shall respect the law and also recognize a responsibility to seek changes in those requirements which are contrary to the best interests of the patient.

IV. A physician shall respect the rights of patients, of colleagues, and of other health professionals, and shall safeguard patient confidence within the constraints of the law.

V. A physician shall continue to study, apply and advance scientific knowledge, make relevant information available to patients, colleagues, and the public, obtain consultation, and use the talents of other health professionals when indicated.

VI. A physician shall, in the provision of appropriate patient care, except in emergencies, be free to choose whom to serve, with whom to associate, and the environment in which to provide medical services.

VII. A physician shall recognize a responsibility to participate in activities contributing to an improved community.

American Nurses Association (ANA) Code for Nurses

1. The nurse provides services with respect for human dignity and the uniqueness of the client, unrestricted by considerations of social or economic status, personal attributes, or the nature of health problems.
2. The nurse safeguards the client's right to privacy by judiciously protecting information of a confidential nature.
3. The nurse acts to safeguard the client and the public when health care and safety are affected by the incompetent, unethical, or illegal practice of any person.
4. The nurse assumes responsibility and accountability for individual nursing judgments and actions.
5. The nurse maintains competence in nursing.
6. The nurse exercises informed judgment and uses individual competence and qualifications as criteria in seeking consultation, accepting responsibilities, and delegating nursing activities to others.
7. The nurse participates in activities that contribute to the ongoing development of the profession's body of knowledge.
8. The nurse participates in the profession's efforts to implement and improve standards of nursing.
9. The nurse participates in the profession's efforts to establish and maintain conditions of employment conducive to high quality nursing care.
10. The nurse participates in the profession's effort to protect the public from misinformation, and misrepresentation and to maintain the integrity of nursing.
11. The nurse collaborates with members of the health profession and other citizens in promoting community and national efforts to meet the health needs of the public.

From "Code for Nurses with Interpretive Statements," © 1985 American Nurses Association, Kansas City, MO. Reprinted with permission.

CODES ON EXPERIMENTATION

Excerpts from the Nuremberg Code on Medical Experiments

The great weight of the evidence before us is to the effect that certain types of medical experiments on human beings, when kept within reasonably well-defined bounds, conform to the ethics of the medical profession generally. The protagonists of the practice of human experimentation justify their views on the basis that such experiments yield results for the good of society that are unprocurable by other methods or means of study. All agree, however, that certain basic principles must be observed in order to satisfy moral, ethical and legal concepts:

1. The voluntary consent of the human subject is absolutely essential. This means that the person involved should have legal capacity to give consent; should be so situated as to be able to exercise free power of choice, without the intervention of any element of force, fraud, deceit, duress, over-reaching, or other ulterior form of constraint or coercion; and should have sufficient knowledge and comprehension of the elements of the subject matter involved as to enable him to make an understanding and enlightened decision. This latter element requires that before the acceptance of an affirmative decision by the experimental subject there should be made known to him the nature, duration, and purpose of the experiment; the method and means by which it is to be conducted; all inconveniences and hazards reasonably to be expected; and the effects upon his health or person which may possibly come from his participation in the experiment.

   The duty and responsibility of ascertaining the quality of the consent rests upon each individual who initiates, directs or engages in the experiment. It is a personal duty and responsibility which may not be delegated to another with impunity.

2. The experiment should be such as to yield fruitful results for the good of society, unprocurable by other methods or means of study, and not random and unnecessary in nature.

3. The experiment should be so designed and based on the results of animal experimentation and a knowledge of the natural history of the disease or other problem under study that the anticipated results will justify the performance of the experiment.

4. The experiment should be so conducted as to avoid all unnecessary physical and mental suffering and injury.

5. No experiment should be conducted where there is an *a priori* reason to believe that death or disabling injury will occur; except, perhaps, in those experiments where the experimental physicians also serve as subjects.

6. The degree of risk to be taken should never exceed that determined by the humanitarian importance of the problem to be solved by the experiment.

7. Proper preparations should be made and adequate facilities provided to protect the experimental subject against even remote possibilities of injury, disability, or death.

8. The experiment should be conducted only by scientifically qualified persons. The highest degree of skill and care should be required through all stages of the experiment of those who conduct or engage in the experiment.

9. During the course of the experiment the human subject should be at liberty to bring the experiment to an end if he has reached the physical or mental state where continuation of the experiment seems to him to be impossible.

10. During the course of the experiment the scientist in charge must be prepared to terminate the experiment at any stage, if he has probable cause to believe, in the exercise of the good faith, superior skill and careful judgment required of him that a continuation of the experiment is likely to result in injury, disability, or death to the experimental subject.

From *Trials of War Criminals before the Nuremberg Military Tribunals*, vol. 2 (1949). Washington, DC: Government Printing Office.

American Medical Association (AMA) Guidelines on Clinical Investigation

2.07 CLINICAL INVESTIGATION. The following guidelines are intended to aid physicians in fulfilling their ethical responsibilities when they engage in the clinical investigation of new drugs and procedures.

(1) A physician may participate in clinical investigation only to the extent that those activities are a part of a systematic program competently designed, under accepted standards of scientific research, to produce data which are scientifically valid and significant.

(2) In conducting clinical investigation, the investigator should demonstrate the same concern and caution for the welfare, safety, and comfort of the person involved as is required of a physician who is furnishing medical care to a patient independent of any clinical investigation.

(3) In clinical investigation primarily for treatment—

A. The physician must recognize that the physician-patient relationship exists and that professional judgment and skill must be exercised in the best interest of the patient.

B. Voluntary written consent must be obtained from the patient, or from his legally authorized representative if the patient lacks the capacity to consent, following: (a) disclosure that the physician intends to use an investigational drug or experimental procedure, (b) a reasonable explanation of the nature of the drug or procedures to be used, risks to be expected, and possible therapeutic benefits, (c) an offer to answer any inquiries concerning the drug or procedure, and (d) a disclosure of alternative drugs or procedures that may be available.

i. In exceptional circumstances and to the extent that disclosure of information concerning the nature of the drug or experimental procedure or risks would be expected to materially affect the health of the patient and would be detrimental to his best interests, such information may be withheld from the patient. In such circumstances, such information shall be disclosed to a responsible relative or friend of the patient where possible.

        ii.   Ordinarily, consent should be in writing, except where the physician deems it necessary to rely upon consent in other than written form because of the physical or emotional state of the patient.

        iii.   Where emergency treatment is necessary, the patient is incapable of giving consent, and no one is available who has authority to act on his behalf, consent is assumed.

(4) In clinical investigation primarily for the accumulation of scientific knowledge—

    A.   Adequate safeguards must be provided for the welfare, safety and comfort of the subject. It is fundamental social policy that the advancement of scientific knowledge must always be secondary to primary concern for the individual.

    B.   Consent, in writing, should be obtained from the subject, or from his legally authorized representative if the subject lacks the capacity to consent, following: (a) a disclosure of the fact that an investigational drug or procedure is to be used, (b) a reasonable explanation of the nature of the procedure to be used and risks to be expected, and (c) an offer to answer any inquiries concerning the drug or procedure.

    C.   Minors or mentally incompetent persons may be used as subjects only if:

        i.   The nature of the investigation is such that mentally competent adults would not be suitable subjects.

        ii.   Consent, in writing, is given by a legally authorized representative of the subject under circumstances in which an informed and prudent adult would reasonably be expected to volunteer himself or his child as a subject.

    D.   No person may be used as a subject against his will.

    E.   The overuse of institutionalized persons in research is an unfair distribution of research risks. Participation is coercive and not voluntary if the participant is subjected to powerful incentives and persuasion. (I, III, V)

2.10 FETAL RESEARCH GUIDELINES. The following guidelines are offered as aids to physicians when they are engaged in fetal research:

    (1)   Physicians may participate in fetal research when their activities are part of a competently designed program, under accepted standards of scientific research, to produce data which are scientifically valid and significant.

    (2)   If appropriate, properly performed clinical studies on animals and nongravid humans should precede any particular fetal research projects.

    (3)   In fetal research projects, the investigator should demonstrate the same care and concern for the fetus as a physician providing fetal care or treatment in a non-research setting.

    (4)   All valid federal or state legal requirements should be followed.

(5) There should be no monetary payment to obtain any fetal material for fetal research projects.

(6) Competent peer review committees, review boards, or advisory boards should be available, when appropriate, to protect against the possible abuses that could arise in such research.

(7) Research on the so called "dead fetus," mascerated fetal material, fetal cells, fetal tissue, or fetal organs should be in accord with state laws on autopsy and state laws on organ transplantation or anatomical gifts.

(8) In fetal research primarily for treatment of the fetus:

    A. Voluntary and informed consent, in writing, should be given by the gravid woman, acting in the best interest of the fetus.

    B. Alternative treatment or methods of care, if any, should be carefully evaluated and fully explained. If simpler and safer treatment is available, it should be pursued.

(9) In research primarily for treatment of the gravid female:

    A. Voluntary and informed consent, in writing, should be given by the patient.

    B. Alternative treatment or methods of care should be carefully evaluated and fully explained to the patient. If simpler and safer treatment is available, it should be pursued.

    C. If possible, the risk to the fetus should be the least possible, consistent with the gravid female's need for treatment.

(10) In fetal research involving a viable fetus, primarily for the accumulation of scientific knowledge:

    A. Voluntary and informed consent, in writing, should be given by the gravid woman under circumstances in which a prudent and informed adult would reasonably be expected to give such consent.

    B. The risk to the fetus imposed by the research should be the least possible.

    C. The purpose of research is the production of data and knowledge which are scientifically significant and which cannot otherwise be obtained.

    D. In this area of research, it is especially important to emphasize that care and concern for the fetus should be demonstrated. There should be no physical abuse of the fetus. (I,III,V)

From *Current Opinions of the Council on Ethical and Judicial Affairs of the American Medical Association,* 1989, Chicago, IL. All rights reserved. Reprinted with permission.

Excerpts from Department of Health and Human Services (HHS) Policy for Protection of Human Research Subjects

§46.101   To what do these regulations apply?

(a)   Except as provided in paragraph (b) of this section, this subpart applies to all research involving human subjects conducted by the Department of Health and Human Services or funded in whole or in part by a Department grant, contract, cooperative agreement or fellowship.

(1)   This includes research conducted by Department employees, except each Principal Operating Component head may adopt such nonsubstantive, procedural modifications as may be appropriate from an administrative standpoint.

(2)   It also includes research conducted or funded by the Department of Health and Human Services outside the United States, but in appropriate circumstances, the Secretary may, under paragraph (e) of this section waive the applicability of some or all of the requirements of these regulations for research of this type.

(b)   Research activities in which the only involvement of human subjects will be in one or more of the following categories are exempt from these regulations unless the research is covered by other subparts of this part:

(1)   Research conducted in established or commonly accepted educational settings, involving normal educational practices, such as (i) research on regular and special education instructional strategies, or (ii) research on the effectiveness of or the comparison among instructional techniques, curricula, or classroom management methods.

(2)   Research involving the use of educational tests (cognitive, diagnostic, aptitude, achievement), if information taken from these sources is recorded in such a manner that subjects cannot be identified, directly or through identifiers linked to the subjects.

(3)   Research involving survey or interview procedures, except where all of the following conditions exist: (i) responses are recorded in such a manner that the human subjects can be identified, directly or through identifiers linked to the subjects, (ii) the subject's responses, if they became known outside the research, could reasonably place the subject at risk of criminal or civil liability or be damaging to the subject's financial standing or employability, and (iii) the research deals with sensitive aspects of the subject's own behavior, such as ille-

gal conduct, drug use, sexual behavior, or use of alcohol. All research involving survey or interview procedures is exempt, without exception, when the respondents are elected or appointed public officials or candidates for public office.

(4) Research involving the observation (including observation by participants) of public behavior, except where all of the following conditions exist: (i) observations are recorded in such a manner that the human subjects can be identified, directly or through identifiers linked to the subjects, (ii) the observations recorded about the individual, if they become known outside the research, could reasonably place the subject at risk of criminal or civil liability or be damaging to the subject's financial standing or employability, and (iii) the research deals with sensitive aspects of the subject's own behavior such as illegal conduct, drug use, sexual behavior, or use of alcohol.

(5) Research involving the collection or study of existing data, documents, records, pathological specimens, or diagnostic specimens, if these sources are publicly available or if the information is recorded by the investigator in such a manner that subjects cannot be identified, directly or through identifiers linked to the subjects.

(6) Unless specifically required by statute (and except to the extent specified in paragraph (i)), research and demonstration projects which are conducted by or subject to the approval of the Department of Health and Human Services, and which are designed to study, evaluate, or otherwise examine: (i) programs under the Social Security Act, or other public benefit or service programs; (ii) procedures for obtaining benefits or services under those programs; (iii) possible changes in or alternatives to those programs or procedures; or (iv) possible changes in methods or levels of payment for benefits or services under those programs.

(c) The Secretary has final authority to determine whether a particular activity is covered by these regulations.

(d) The Secretary may require that specific research activities or classes of research activities conducted or funded by the Department, but not otherwise covered by these regulations, comply with some or all of these regulations.

(e) The Secretary may also waive applicability of these regulations to specific research activities or classes of research activities, otherwise covered by these regulations. Notices of these actions will be published in the *Federal Register* as they occur.

(f) No individual may receive Department funding for research covered by these regulations unless the individual is affiliated with or sponsored by an institution which assumes responsibility for the research under an assurance satisfying the requirements of this part, or the individual makes other arrangements with the Department.

(g) Compliance with these regulations will in no way render inapplicable pertinent federal, state, or local laws or regulations.

(h) Each subpart of these regulations contains a separate section describing to what the subpart applies. Research which is covered by more than one subpart shall comply with all applicable subparts.

(i) If, following review of proposed research activities that are exempt from these regulations under paragraph (b)(6), the Secretary determines that a research or demonstration project presents a danger to the physical, mental, or emotional well-being of a participant or subject of the research or demonstration project, then federal funds may not be expended for such a project without the written, informed consent of each participant or subject.

§46.110   Expedited review procedures for certain kinds of research involving no more than minimal risk, and for minor changes in approved research.

(a)   The Secretary has established, and published in the *Federal Register*, a list of categories of research that may be reviewed by the IRB through an expedited review procedure. The list will be amended, as appropriate, through periodic republication in the *Federal Register*.

(b)   An IRB may review some or all of the research appearing on the list through an expedited review procedure, if the research involves no more than minimal risk. The IRB may also use the expedited review procedure to review minor changes in previously approved research during the period for which approval is authorized. Under an expedited review procedure, the review may be carried out by the IRB chairperson or by one or more experienced reviewers designated by the chairperson from among members of the IRB. In reviewing the research, the reviewers may exercise all of the authorities of the IRB except that the reviewers may not disapprove the research. A research activity may be disapproved only after review in accordance with the non-expedited procedure set forth on § 46.108(b).

(c)   Each IRB which uses an expedited review procedure shall adopt a method for keeping all members advised of research proposals which have been approved under the procedure.

(d)   The Secretary may restrict, suspend, or terminate an institution's or IRB's use of the expedited review procedure when necessary to protect the rights or welfare of subjects.

§46.111   Criteria for IRB approval of research.

(a)   In order to approve research covered by these regulations the IRB shall determine that all of the following requirements are satisfied:

(1)   Risks to subjects are minimized: (i) By using procedures which are consistent with sound research design and which do not unnecessarily expose subjects to risk, and (ii) whenever appropriate, by using procedures already being performed on the subjects for diagnostic or treatment purposes.

(2)   Risks to subjects are reasonable in relation to anticipated benefits, if any, to subjects, and the importance of the knowledge that may reasonably be expected to result. In evaluating risks and benefits, the IRB should consider only those risks and benefits that may result from the research (as distinguished from risks and benefits of therapies subjects would receive even if not participating in the research). The IRB should not consider possible long-range effects of applying knowledge gained in the research (for example, the possible effects of the research on public policy) as among those research risks that fall within the purview of its responsibility.

(3)   Selection of subjects is equitable. In making this assessment the IRB

should take into account the purposes of the research and the setting in which the research will be conducted.

(4) Informed consent will be sought from each prospective subject or the subject's legally authorized representative, in accordance with, and to the extent required by § 46.116.

(5) Informed consent will be appropriately documented, in accordance with, and to the extent required by § 46.117.

(6) Where appropriate, the research plan makes adequate provision for monitoring the data collected to insure the safety of subjects.

(7) Where appropriate, there are adequate provisions to protect the privacy of subjects and to maintain the confidentiality of data.

(b) Where some or all of the subjects are likely to be vulnerable to coercion or undue influence, such as persons with acute or severe physical or mental illness, or persons who are economically or educationally disadvantaged, appropriate additional safeguards have been included in the study to protect the rights and welfare of these subjects.

§46.116   General requirements for informed consent.

Except as provided elsewhere in this or other subparts, no investigator may involve a human being as a subject in research covered by these regulations unless the investigator has obtained the legally effective informed consent of the subject or the subject's legally authorized representative. An investigator shall seek such consent only under circumstances that provide the prospective subject or the representative sufficient opportunity to consider whether or not to participate and that minimize the possibility of coercion or undue influence. The information that is given to the subject or the representative shall be in language understandable to the subject or the representative. No informed consent, whether oral or written, may include any exculpatory language through which the subject or the representative is made to waive or appear to waive any of the subject's legal rights, or releases or appears to release the investigator, the sponsor, the institution or its agents from liability for negligence.

(a) Basic elements of informed consent. Except as provided in paragraph (c) or (d) of this section, in seeking informed consent the following information shall be provided to each subject:

(1) A statement that the study involves research, an explanation of the purposes of the research and the expected duration of the subject's participation, a description of the procedures to be followed, and identification of any procedures which are experimental;

(2) A description of any reasonably foreseeable risks or discomforts to the subject;

(3) A description of any benefits to the subject or to others which may reasonably be expected from the research;

(4) A disclosure of appropriate alternative procedures or courses of treatment, if any, that might be advantageous to the subject;

(5) A statement describing the extent, if any, to which confidentiality of records identifying the subject will be maintained;

(6) For research involving more than minimal risk, an explanation as to

whether any compensation and an explanation as to whether any medical treatments are available if injury occurs and, if so, what they consist of, or where further information may be obtained;

(7) An explanation of whom to contact for answers to pertinent questions about the research and research subjects' rights, and whom to contact in the event of a research-related injury to the subject; and

(8) A statement that participation is voluntary, refusal to participate will involve no penalty or loss of benefits to which the subject is otherwise entitled, and the subject may discontinue participation at any time without penalty or loss of benefits to which the subject is otherwise entitled.

(b) Additional elements of informed consent. When appropriate, one or more of the following elements of information shall also be provided to each subject:

(1) A statement that the particular treatment or procedure may involve risks to the subject (or to the embryo or fetus, if the subject is or may become pregnant) which are currently unforeseeable;

(2) Anticipated circumstances under which the subject's participation may be terminated by the investigator without regard to the subject's consent;

(3) Any additional costs to the subject that may result from participation in the research;

(4) The consequences of a subject's decision to withdraw from the research and procedures for orderly termination of participation by the subject;

(5) A statment that significant new findings developed during the course of the research which may relate to the subject's willingness to continue participation will be provided to the subject; and

(6) The approximate number of subjects involved in the study.

(c) An IRB may approve a consent procedure which does not include, or which alters, some or all of the elements of informed consent set forth above, or waive the requirement to obtain informed consent provided the IRB finds and documents that:

(1) The reserach or demonstration project is to be conducted by or subject to the approval of state or local government officials and is designed to study, evaluate, or otherwise examine: (i) programs under the Social Security Act, or other public benefit or service programs; (ii) procedures for obtaining benefits or services under those programs; (iii) possible changes in or alternatives to those programs or procedures; or (iv) possible changes in methods or levels of payment for benefits or services under those programs; and

(2) The research could not practicably be carried out without the waiver or alteration.

(d) An IRB may approve a consent procedure which does not include, or which alters, some or all of the elements of informed consent set forth above, or waive the requirements to obtain informed consent provided the IRB finds and documents that:

(1) The research involves no more than minimal risk to the subjects;

(2) The waiver or alteration will not adversely affect the rights and welfare of the subjects;

(3) The research could not practicably be carried out without the waiver or alteration; and

(4)   Whenever appropriate, the subjects will be provided with additional pertinent information after participation.

(e)   The informed consent requirements in these regulations are not intended to preempt any applicable federal, state, or local laws which require additional information to be disclosed in order for informed consent to be legally effective.

(f)   Nothing in these regulations is intended to limit the authority of a physician to provide emergency medical care, to the extent the physician is permitted to do so under applicable federal, state, or local law.

§46.117   Documentation of informed consent.

(a)   Except as provided in paragraph (c) of this section, informed consent shall be documented by the use of a written consent form approved by the IRB and signed by the subject or the subject's legally authorized representative. A copy shall be given to the person signing the form.

(b)   Except as provided in paragraph (c) of this section, the consent form may be either of the following:

(1)   A written consent document that embodies the elements of informed consent required by § 46.116. This form may be read to the subject or the subject's legally authorized representative, but in any event, the investigator shall give either the subject or the representative adequate opportunity to read it before it is signed; or

(2)   A "short form" written consent document stating that the elements of informed consent required by § 46.116 have been presented orally to the subject or the subject's legally authorized representative. When this method is used, there shall be a witness to the oral presentation. Also, the IRB shall approve a written summary of what is to be said to the subject or the representative. Only the short form itself is to be signed by the subject or the representative. However, the witness shall sign both the short form and a copy of the summary, and the person actually obtaining consent shall sign a copy of the summary. A copy of the summary shall be given to the subject or the representative, in addition to a copy of the "short form."

(c)   An IRB may waive the requirement for the investigator to obtain a signed consent form for some or all subjects if it finds either:

(1)   That the only record linking the subject and the research would be the consent document and the principal risk would be potential harm resulting from a breach of confidentiality. Each subject will be asked whether the subject wants documentation linking the subject with the research, and the subject's wishes will govern; or

(2)   That the research presents no more than minimal risk of harm to subjects and involves no procedures for which written consent is normally required outside of the research context.

In cases where the documentation requirement is waived, the IRB may require the investigator to provide subjects with a written statement regarding the research.

From Department of Health and Human Resources, "Basic HHS Policy for Protection of Human Research Subjects," 46 CFR, pp. 98 et seq. (1981, as modified). The following regulations have been omitted: experimenting on fetuses, pregnant women, and human *in vitro* fertilization; biomedical and behavioral research involving prisoners as subjects; and protections for children as subjects in research.

∞

BIBLIOGRAPHY

Books

Beauchamp, Tom L., and James F. Childress. *Principles of Biomedical Ethics*. 3rd ed. New York: Oxford University Press, 1989.

Cranford, Ronald E., and A. Edward Doudera, eds. *Institutional Ethics Committees and Health Care Decision Making*. Ann Arbor: Health Administration Press, 1984.

Darr, Kurt. *Ethics for Health Services Managers*. Vol. 4, *Case Studies in Health Administration*. Chicago: Foundation of the American College of Hospital Administrators, 1985.

DeGeorge, Richard T. *Business Ethics*. 3rd ed. New York: Macmillan, 1990.

Engelhardt, H. Tristam, Jr. *The Foundations of Bioethics*. New York: Oxford University Press, 1986.

Fletcher, John C., Norman Quist, and Albert R. Johnson. *Ethics Consultation in Health Care*. Ann Arbor: Health Administration Press, 1989.

Frankena, William K. *Ethics*. 2nd ed. Englewood Cliffs, NJ: Prentice Hall, 1973.

Pellegrino, Edmund D., and David C. Thomasma. *For the Patient's Good: The Restoration of Beneficence in Health Care*. New York: Oxford University Press, 1988.

President's Commission for the Study of Ethical Problems in Medicine and Biomedical and Behavioral Research. Reports on various topics: *Summing Up; Compensating for Research Injuries*, 2 vols.; *Deciding to Forego Life-Sustaining Treatment; Defining Death; Implementing Human Research Regulations; Making Health Care Decisions*, 2 vols.; *Protecting Human Subjects; Screening and Counseling for Genetic Conditions; Securing Access to Health Care*, 3 vols.; *Splicing Life;* and *Whistleblowing in Biomedical Research*. Washington, DC: Government Printing Office: 1980–1983.

Veatch, Robert M. *A Theory of Medical Ethics*. New York: Basic Books, 1981.

Wing, Kenneth R. *The Law and the Public's Health*. 2nd ed. Ann Arbor: Health Administration Press, 1985.

Other Publications

Aaron, Henry J., and W. B. Schwartz. "Hospital Cost Control: A Bitter Pill to Swallow." *Harvard Business Review 63* (March/April 1985: 160–167.

Ackerman, Terrence F. "Why Doctors Should Intervene." *Hastings Center Report 12* (August 1982): 14–17.

Aday, Lu Ann, and Ronald M. Anderson. "Equity of Access to Medical Care: A Conceptual and Empirical Overview." *Medical Care 19* (12 Suppl.) (December 1981): 4–27.

American College of Healthcare Executives. "Code of Ethics." Chicago: American College of Healthcare Executives, 1987.

Angell, Marcia. "Cost Containment and the Physician." *Journal of the American Medical Association 254* (September 1985): 1203–1207.

Angell, Marcia. "Respecting the Autonomy of Competent Patients." *New England Journal of Medicine 310* (April 1984): 1115–1116.

Annas, George J. "CPR: When the Beat Should Stop." *Hastings Center Report 12* (October 1982): 30–31.

Annas, George J. "Do Feeding Tubes Have More Rights than Patients?" *Hastings Center Report 11* (February 1986): 26–32.

Annas, George J. "Who to Call When the Doctor is Sick." *Hastings Center Report 8* (December 1978): 18–20.

"Applied Ethics: A Strategy for Fostering Professional Responsibility." *Carnegie Quarterly 28* (Spring/Summer 1980): 1–7.

Arras, John D. "Health Care Vouchers and the Rhetoric of Equity." *Hastings Center Report 11* (August 1981): 29–39.

Bernat, James L., Charles M. Culver, and Bernard Gert. "Defining Death in Theory and Practice." *Hastings Center Report 12* (February 1982): 5–9.

Blake, David C. "State Interests in Terminating Medical Treatment." *Hastings Center Report 19* (May/June 1989): 5–13.

Brody, Howard. "Transparency: Informed Consent in Primary Care." *Hastings Center Report 19* (September/October 1989): 5–9.

Brozovich, John P. "Managing Change Through Values." *Healthcare Executive* (March/April 1986): 45–47.

Callahan, Daniel. "How Technology is Reframing the Abortion Debate." *Hastings Center Report 16* (February 1986): 33–42.

Callahan, Daniel. "On Feeding the Dying." *Hastings Center Report 13* (October 1983): 22.

Callahan, Daniel. "Terminating Treatment: Age as a Standard." *Hastings Center Report 17* (October/November 1987): 21–25.

Caplan, Arthur L. "Kidneys, Ethics, and Politics: Policy Lessons of the ESRD Experience." *Journal of Health, Politics and Law 6* (Fall 1981): 488–503.

Childress, James F. "The Place of Autonomy in Bioethics." *Hastings Center Report 20* (January/February 1990): 12–17.

Cleveland, Henry C., III, and Barbara L. Crawford. "When Physicians Refuse to Treat Patients with AIDS." *Trustee 41* (March 1988): 18–19.

Clouser, K. Danner. "Life-Support Systems: Some Moral Reflections." *American College of Surgeons Bulletin 68* (June 1983): 12–17.

Cohen, Cynthia B., ed. "Ethics Committees." *Hastings Center Report 18* (August/September 1988): 23–28.

Cohen, Cynthia B., ed. "Ethics Committees." *Hastings Center Report 19* (January/February 1989): 19–24.

Cohen, Cynthia B., ed. "Ethics Committees." *Hastings Center Report 19* (September/October 1989): 21–26.

Curtis, Joy. "Multidisciplinary Input on Institutional Ethics Committees: A Nursing Perspective." *Quality Review Bulletin 10* (July 1984): 199–202.

Darr, Kurt. "Administrative Ethics and the Health Services Manager." *Hospital & Health Services Administration 29* (March/April 1984): 120–136.

Darr, Kurt, Beaufort Longest, Jr., and Jonathon Rakich. "The Ethical Imperative in Health Services Governance and Management." *Hospital & Health Services Administration 31* (March/April 1986): 53–66.

Detsky, Allan S., S.C. Stricker, and A.G. Mulley. "Prognosis, Survival, and the Expenditure of Hospital Resources for Patients in an Intensive Care Unit." *New England Journal of Medicine 305* (September 1981): 667–672.

Dine, Deborah Denaro. "Ethics." *Modern Healthcare 18* (October 1988): 22–30.

Dolenc, Danielle, A., and Charles J. Dougherty. "DRGs: The Counterrevolution in Financing Health Care." *Hastings Center Report 15* (June 1985): 19–29.

Dougherty, Charles J. "Cost Containment, DRGs, and the Ethics of Health Care." *Hastings Center Report 19* (January/February 1989): 5–11.

Dunlop, George R. "President's Commission Offers Guidelines on Life-Support Therapy." *American College of Surgeons Bulletin 68* (June 1983): 8–11.

Dworkin, Gerald. "Taking Risks, Assessing Responsibility." *Hastings Center Report 11* (October 1981): 26–39.

Emery, Danielle Dolenc, and Lawrence J. Schneiderman. "Cost-Effectiveness Analysis in Health Care." *Hastings Center Report 19* (July/August 1989): 8–13.

Engelhardt, H. Tristram. "Allocating Scarce Medical Resources and the Availability of Organ Transplantation." *New England Journal of Medicine 311* (July 1984): 66–71.

Ertel, Paul Y., and R. Van Harrison. "Ethical and Operational Issues Concerning DRGs and the Prospective Payment System." *Topics in Health Care Management 4* (March 1984): 10–31.

"Ethics Committees: How Are They Doing?" *Hastings Center Report 16* (June 1986): 9–24.

Evans, Andrew, and Baruch Brody. "The Do-Not-Resuscitate Order in Teaching Hospitals." *Journal of the American Medical Association 293* (April 1985): 2236–2239.

Faden, Ruth R., C. Becker, and C. Lewis. "Disclosure of Information to Patients in Medical Care." *Medical Care 19* (July 1981): 718–733.

Fost, Norman, and Ronald E. Cranford. "Hospital Ethics Committees, Administrative Aspects." *Journal of the American Medical Association 253* (May 1985): 2687–2692.

Freedman, Benjamin. "One Philosopher's Experience on an Ethics Committee." *Hastings Center Report 11* (April 1981): 20–22.

Glazer, Myron. "Ten Whistleblowers and How They Fared." *Hastings Center Report 13* (December 1983): 33–41.

Gostin, Lawrence. "HIV-Infected Physicians and the Practice of Seriously Invasive Procedures." *Hastings Center Report 19* (January/February 1989): 32–39.

Gray, Bradford H. "Complexities of Informed Consent." *Annals of the American Academy 437* (May 1978): 37–48.

Gregory, Charles L. "Ethics: A Management Tool?" *Hospital & Health Services Administration 29* (March/April 1984): 102–119.

Grodin, M.A., and Betal Zaharoff. "A 12-Year Audit of IRB Decisions." *Quality Review Bulletin 12* (March 1986): 82–86.

Hardin, Garrett. "Limited World, Limited Rights." *Society 17* (May/June 1980): 5–8.

Hiller, Marc D. "Ethics and Health Care Administration: Issues in Education and Practice." *Journal of Health Administration Education 2* (Spring 1984): 147–192.

Hofmann, Paul B. "Business Ethics: Not an Oxymoron." *Healthcare Executive 2* (September/October 1987): 22–24.

Jonsen, Albert R. "Watching the Doctor." *New England Journal of Medicine 308* (June 1983): 1531–1535.

Judicial Council. "Guidelines for Ethics Committees in Health Care Institutions." *Journal of the American Medical Association 253* (May 1985): 2698–2699.

Kapp, Marshall B. "Legal and Ethical Implications of Health Care Reimbursement by Diagnosis-Related Groups." *Law, Medicine and Health Care 12* (December 1984): 245–253.

Levine, Carol. "Ethics Committees: Trend for Troubling Times." *Hospital Medical Staff 12* (June 1983): 2–8.

Levine, Carol. "Questions and (Some Very Tentative) Answers About Hospital Ethics Committees." *Hastings Center Report 14* (June 1984): 9–12.

Lipton, Helene. "Do-Not-Resuscitate Decisions in a Community Hospital: Implications for Quality Care." *Quality Review Bulletin 13* (July 1987): 226–231.

Lo, Bernard, T.A. Raffin, and N.H. Cohen. "Ethical Dilemmas About Intensive Care for Patients with AIDS." *Reviews of Infectious Diseases 9* (November/December 1987): 1163–1167.

Longo, Daniel, M. Warren, and J.S. Roberts. "Extent of DNR Policies Varies Across Healthcare Settings." *Health Progress 69* (June 1988): 66–73.

Lynn, Joanne, and James F. Childress. "Must Patients Always be Given Food and Water?" *Hastings Center Report 13* (October 1983): 17–21.

Macklin, Ruth. "Dilemmas of Informed Consent for Surgery." *American College of Surgeons Bulletin 67* (July 1982): 6–9.

McCullough, Laurence B. "Moral Dilemmas and Economic Realities." *Hospital & Health Services Administration 30* (September/October 1985): 63–75.

McPhail, Aileen, S. Moore, and J. O'Connor. "One Hospital's Experience with a 'Do-not-resuscitate' Policy." *CMA Journal 127* (October 1981): 830–836.

Medical Consultants on the Diagnosis of Death to the President's Commission for the Study of Ethical Problems in Medicine and Biomedical and Behavioral Research. "Guidelines for the Determination of Death," *Journal of the American Medical Association 246* (November 1981): 2184–2186.

Mehlman, Maxwell J. "Encouraging Donation of Organs for Transplantation by Requiring Request." *Health Matrix 5* (Summer 1987): 35–38.

Mooney, Gavin H. "Cost–Benefit Analysis and Medical Ethics." *Journal of Medical Ethics 6* (December 1980): 177–179.

Morreim, E. Haavi. "The MD and the DRG." *Hastings Center Report 15* (June 1985): 30–38.

Murray, Thomas H. "The Final, Anticlimactic Rule on Baby Doe." *Hastings Center Report 15* (June 1985): 5–9.

Nolan, Kathleen. "In Death's Shadow: The Meanings of Withholding Resuscitation." *Hastings Center Report 17* (October/November 1987): 9–14.

Powderly, Kathleen E., and Elaine Smith. "The Impact of DRGs on Health Care Workers and Their Clients." *Hastings Center Report 19* (January/February 1989): 16–18.

Rachels, James. "Can Ethics Provide Answers?" *Hastings Center Report 10* (June 1980): 32–40.

Rasinski, Dorothy C. "Ethics Committees in Hospitals: Alternative Structures and Responsibilities." *Quality Review Bulletin 10* (March 1984): 62–64.

Relman, Arnold S. "AIDS: The Emerging Ethical Dilemma." *Hastings Center Report 15* (August 1985): 1–7.

Relman, Arnold S. "Dealing with Conflicts of Interest." *New England Journal of Medicine 313* (September 1985): 749–751.

Rhoden, Nancy K. "A Compromise on Abortion?" *Hastings Center Report 19* (July/August 1989): 32–37.

Robertson, John A. "Ethics Committees in Hospitals: Alternative Structures and Responsibilities." *Quality Review Bulletin 10* (January 1984): 6–10.

Rosner, Fred. "Hospital Medical Ethics Committees: A Review of Their Development." *Journal of the American Medical Association 253* (May 1985): 2693–2697.

Ross, Judith Wilson, and Deborah Pugh. "Limited Cardiopulmonary Resuscitation: The Ethics of Partial Codes." *Quality Review Bulletin 14* (January 1988): 4–8.

Rovers, John P. "The Ethics of Biomedical Research in Humans." *Health Matrix 5* (Summer 1987): 21–25.

Seiden, Dena J. "Ethics for Hospital Administrators." *Hospital & Health Services Administration 28* (March/April 1983): 81–89.

Stein, Kathleen. "Last Rights." *Omni 9* (September 1987): 59.

Steinbock, Bonnie. "Recovery from Persistent Vegetative State?: The Case of Carrie Coons." *Hastings Center Report 19* (July/August 1989): 14–15.

Thomasma, David C. "Hospitals' Ethical Responsibilities as Technology, Regulation Grow." *Hospital Progress 63* (December 1982): 74–79.

Thomasma, David C. "The Range of Euthanasia." *American College of Surgeons Bulletin 73* (August 1988): 4–13.

Tomlinson, Tom, and Howard Brody. "Ethics and Communication in Do-not-resuscitate Orders." *New England Journal of Medicine 318* (January 1988): 43–46.

U.S. Department of Health and Human Services. *Basic HHS Policy for Protection of Human Research Subjects.* 46 CFR, 98 et seq. (1981, as modified).

U.S. Department of Health and Human Services, Office of Human Development Services. *Child Abuse and Neglect Prevention and Treatment Program* (Final Rule); and *Model Guidelines for Health Care Providers to Establish Infant Care Review Committees* (Notice). 45 CFR Part 1340 (April 15, 1985).

Veatch, Robert M. "DRGs and the Ethical Allocation of Resources." *Hastings Center Report 16* (June 1986): 32–40.

Veatch, Robert M. "Professional Ethics: New Principles for Physicians?" *Hastings Center Report 10* (June 1980): 16–19.

Veatch, Robert M. "Protecting Human Subjects: The Federal Government Steps Back." *Hastings Report Center 11* (June 1981): 9–14.

Veatch, Robert M. "What it Means to Be Dead." *Hastings Center Report 12* (December 1982): 45.

Weiss, Rick. "Forbidding Fruits of Fetal-Cell Research." *Science News 134* (November 1988): 296–298.

Weitz, Rose. "The Interview as Legacy: A Social Scientist Confronts AIDS." *Hastings Center Report 17* (June 1987): 21–23.

Wielk, Carol A. "Human Experimentation: Issues Before the Hospital Administrator." *Hospital & Health Services Administration 22* (Summer 1977): 4–25.

Wigodsky, Herman S. "New Regulations, New Responsibilities for Institutions." *Hastings Center Report 11* (June 1981): 12–14.

Wolf, Susan M., ed. "The Persistent Problem of PVS." *Hastings Center Report 18* (February/March 1988): 26–47.

Younger, Stuart J. "Do-Not-Resuscitate Orders: No Longer Secret, But Still a Problem." *Hastings Center Report 17* (February 1987): 24–33.

Zimmerman, Jack E., W.A. Knaus, and S.M. Sharpe. "The Use and Implications of Do-Not-Resuscitate Orders in Intensive Care Units." *Journal of the American Medical Association 255* (January 1986): 351–356.

∞

INDEX